COMPLICATIONS OF
Urologic
Laparoscopic
Surgery

COMPLICATIONS OF
Urologic Laparoscopic Surgery
RECOGNITION, MANAGEMENT AND PREVENTION

EDITED BY

SANJAY RAMAKUMAR
University of Arizona Health Sciences Center
Tucson, Arizona, U.S.A.

THOMAS JARRETT
Johns Hopkins Medical Institutions
Baltimore, Maryland, U.S.A.

informa
healthcare

New York London

First published in 2005 by Taylor & Francis Group, 6000 Broken Sound Parkway NW, Suite 300, Boca Raton, FL 33487-2742, USA.

This edition published in 2010 by Informa Healthcare, Telephone House, 69-77 Paul Street, London EC2A 4LQ, UK.

Simultaneously published in the USA by Informa Healthcare, 52 Vanderbilt Avenue, 7th Floor, New York, NY 10017, USA.

Informa Healthcare is a trading division of Informa UK Ltd. Registered Office: 37–41 Mortimer Street, London W1T 3JH, UK. Registered in England and Wales number 1072954.

A CIP record for this book is available from the British Library.

Library of Congress Cataloging-in-Publication Data available on application

ISBN-13: 9780824726591

Orders may be sent to: Informa Healthcare, Sheepen Place, Colchester, Essex CO3 3LP, UK
Telephone: +44 (0)20 7017 5540
Email: CSDhealthcarebooks@informa.com
Website: http://informahealthcarebooks.com/

For corporate sales please contact: CorporateBooksIHC@informa.com
For foreign rights please contact: RightsIHC@informa.com
For reprint permissions please contact: PermissionsIHC@informa.com

Preface

Laparoscopy has made a significant impact on the surgical management of disease. Advances in technology such as the CCD camera, improved optics, computerized systems, and smaller instrumentation have expanded applications from diagnostic procedures to advanced ablative and reconstructive surgery. Urologists were well positioned for this revolution because of the endoscopic skills already acquired with transurethral surgery. Surgeons now have an increasing awareness of the impact an operation has on a patient and that minimizing morbidity and decreasing convalescence are essential to patient care. All the surgical principles such as cancer control, hemostasis, and asepsis are maintained with the patient returning to normal life significantly faster and with less suffering.

Minimally invasive surgery, however, has some drawbacks, which may be responsible for its slow acceptance in all disciplines. Training in these techniques is difficult and only recently have training programs incorporated laparoscopic surgery as a key training component. Surgeons who completed training before the laparoscopic era may find it difficult to spend the time and effort required for safe laparoscopic surgery. Also, longer operating times associated with laparoscopic surgery can be a disincentive to this approach. Despite this, the surgical community continues to pursue advanced laparoscopic skills for the benefit of their patients.

An integral component of laparoscopic training is a keen understanding of the potential pitfalls that may arise. Although the magnification provided with laparoscopy provides better visualization, complications are still difficult to recognize owing to the sometimes unfamiliar anatomy, decreased tactile feedback, 3-D vision and ability to only visualize small portions of the surgical field at a given time. Furthermore, the distance between operator and surgical field prevents a surgeon from "placing one's hands in the wound and saving the day."

The laparoscopist must develop a "sixth sense" and anticipate problems. This concept is not different from open surgery, but the clinical clues during the operation are different and need to be understood. When a complication does occur, open conversion is not always necessary and laparoscopic techniques to correct a problem exist. Laparoscopic procedures have also seen a unique set of complications, perhaps a reflection of the learning curve or a different approach to the operative site. Understanding these principles is the key to successful prevention strategies and good outcomes.

Rather than subdividing this text by procedure, we chose to focus on broad categories of complications seen with laparoscopic urologic surgery, their recognition, management, and prevention. Finally, this manual can provide the reader an easy reference than can be incorporated into any laparoscopic training program as well as a step-by-step guide to recognizing and managing difficult situations for surgeons already performing minimally invasive surgery.

Sanjay Ramakumar
Thomas Jarrett

Contents

Contributors

Timothy D. Averch   The University of Pittsburgh Medical Center, Kaufmann Medical Building, Pittsburgh, Pennsylvania, U.S.A.

Jay T. Bishoff   Endourology Section, Department of Urology, Wilford Hall Medical Center, Lackland Air Force Base, Texas, U.S.A.

Jeffrey A. Cadeddu   The Clinical Center for Minimally Invasive Urologic Cancer Treatment, Department of Urology, University of Texas, Southwestern Medical Center at Dallas, Dallas, Texas, U.S.A.

David Y. Chan   The James Buchanan Brady Urological Institute, Johns Hopkins Medical Institutions, Baltimore, Maryland, U.S.A.

George K. Chow   Department of Urology, Mayo Clinic, Rochester, Minnesota, U.S.A.

Peter Colegrove   University of Arizona Health Sciences Center, Tucson, Arizona, U.S.A.

David C. Cuellar   The University of Pittsburgh Medical Center, Kaufmann Medical Building, Pittsburgh, Pennsylvania, U.S.A.

Joseph J. Del Pizzo   James Buchanan Brady Urological Foundation, The New York-Presbyterian Hospital, University Hospital of Cornell, New York, New York, U.S.A.

Oscar Fugita   Division of Surgery, University of São Paulo, São Paulo, Brazil

Matthew T. Gettman   Department of Urology, Mayo Clinic, Rochester, Minnesota, U.S.A.

Thomas Jarrett   Division of Urology, Johns Hopkins Medical Institutions, Baltimore, Maryland, U.S.A.

Benjamin R. Lee   Department of Urology, Long Island Jewish Medical Center, New Hyde Park, New York, U.S.A.

Robert Marcovich   Department of Urology, University of Texas Health Sciences Center, San Antonio, Texas, U.S.A.

Kenneth Ogan   The Clinical Center for Minimally Invasive Urologic Cancer Treatment, Department of Urology, University of Texas, Southwestern Medical Center at Dallas, Dallas, Texas, U.S.A.

Eugene Park   Urological Associates of Southern Arizona, P.C, Tucson, Arizona, U.S.A.

Timothy M. Philips   Endourology Section, Department of Urology, Wilford Hall Medical Center, Lackland Air Force Base, Texas, U.S.A.

Sanjay Ramakumar   University of Arizona Health Sciences Center, Tucson, Arizona, U.S.A.

R. Ernest Sosa   The New York Presbyterian Hospital, Joan and Sanford I. Weill Medical College, New York, New York, U.S.A.

Li-Ming Su   James Buchanan Brady Urological Institute, Johns Hopkins Medical Institutions, Baltimore, Maryland, U.S.A.

Jon Varkarakis   Second Department of Urology, University of Athens, Athens, Greece

Ozgur Yaycioglu   Department of Urology, Baskent University School of Medicine, Adana Clinic & Research Center, Adana, Turkey

Paul Yurkanin   Southern Arizona Urologic Oncology, Tucson, Arizona, U.S.A.

1

Anesthetic Considerations/ Complications

DAVID C. CUELLAR and TIMOTHY D. AVERCH

The University of Pittsburgh Medical Center,
Kaufmann Medical Building, Pittsburgh,
Pennsylvania, U.S.A.

Inherent in surgical procedures is the consideration of risks of anesthesia. Concerns specific to laparoscopic surgery including patient positioning need to be understood and addressed prior to undertaking these procedures. Specifically, the effects of pneumoperitoneum and carbon dioxide, alterations in renal physiology, and changes to the circulatory system will be addressed herein.

Consideration must always be given for carbon dioxide absorption during laparoscopy. Hypercarbia can result from increased CO_2 load caused by transperitoneal or subcutaneous absorption of insufflated CO_2 (1–3) with significant effects on acid–base balance and hemodynamic stability (4–7). Most of the increase in $PaCO_2$ occurs in the first 15 min and remains stable (8), but can be more pronounced with prolonged insufflation time (9–13), especially during the first 2 hr of insufflation (14), with increased insufflation pressures (15–17), and with subcutaneous emphysema (14,18–20). Carbon dioxide diffusion into body tissues is greater during extraperitoneal than intraperitoneal CO_2 insufflation (14,21,22). Although some studies have demonstrated a greater increase in partial pressure of arterial carbon dioxide with obese patients undergoing laparoscopic surgery (17), others have shown the contrary (14). The effect of the location of the operative site on carbon dioxide absorption has also been shown to be significant with pelvic laparoscopy demonstrating less absorption than renal laparoscopy (14).

The clinical significance of increased CO_2 absorption is unclear as there are rarely cardiopulmonary complications related to hypercapnea. To minimize complications, one should avoid insufflation pressures above 15 mmHg if possible and be more alert with retroperitoneal CO_2 insufflation, with subcutaneous emphysema, with long insufflation times, during renal laparoscopy, and in the obese patient. It has been demonstrated that an insufflation pressure of 20 mmHg can be maintained in most patients with adjustments in minute ventilation (23). Arterial CO_2 should be monitored closely intra- and postoperatively in these situations until it returns to baseline.

In patients with severe pulmonary compromise who are at risk for severe acidosis, gasless laparoscopy and insufflation with helium as an alternative have been described. Studies have shown a decrease in the acidosis compared to carbon dioxide (12). This may allow laparoscopic procedures in patients felt to be at too high risk due to underlying pulmonary compromise.

Gas embolism is a rare but severe complication of laparoscopic surgery. It may be due to direct puncture of a major vessel or pressure-forced entry of carbon dioxide into a venous plexus (24). The mixture of gas and blood affects the pulmonary vasculature leading to pulmonary hypertension and fatal right ventricular failure. Decrease in venous return leads to compromise of cardiac output and collapse. A sudden drop in PCO_2 is a strong indicator of air embolism. When CO_2 is used for insufflation, however, the PCO_2 may not change or it may increase. Other warning signs are a significant decrease in SpO_2, heart rate, and blood pressure, along with a cardiac arrhythmia and total collapse. Transesophageal ECHO has been utilized to monitor for gas embolism during laparoscopic surgery both in the porcine model (25) and in humans (26). Although sensitive, it detects many clinically insignificant emboli.

If gas embolism is suspected, the procedure should be terminated with immediate release of CO_2, high-fraction-inspired O_2 ventilation, left lateral decubitus positioning (Durant's position), and pericardial thumps or cardiac massage. Aspiration of the gas via a central venous catheter (24) and cardiopulmonary bypass has also been reported as treatments (27). Due to its high solubility, CO_2 embolism is fortunately rare (28). The risk appears to be higher with retroperitoneal rather than peritoneal laparoscopy because of the limited and nonexpansible retroperitoneal space. Prevention measures include limiting the insufflation pressure, especially with retroperitoneoscopy.

Subcutaneous emphysema from CO_2 insufflation is a known complication of laparoscopic surgery. It can usually be detected on physical exam or chest x-ray. It was documented by CT scan after uncomplicated laparoscopic cholecystectomy in 56% of patients studied, all of who were asymptomatic (29). Clinically significant cases occur in 2–12 per 1000 cases and usually resolve spontaneously within 24 hr (30). Unlike intraperitoneal placement of CO_2, significant subcutaneous emphysema may lead to significant changes in pH and $PaCO_2$ as demonstrated in the porcine model (31). This difference between subcutaneous and intraperitoneal CO_2 is thought to be due to the relative ease of removal of intraperitoneal CO_2 via the trocar ports, whereas subcutaneous CO_2 is absorbed and must be removed via the lungs. Patients who develop significant subcutaneous emphysema following laparoscopic surgery should be closely monitored until pH and $PaCO_2$ return to baseline.

Another important consideration with laparoscopic surgery is alterations in renal physiology. Changes have been shown to occur with prolonged intraabdominal CO_2 insufflation, especially in high-risk patients with cardiovascular, hemodynamic, and renal dysfunction. This cause is likely multifactorial and includes decrease in cardiac output, renovascular compression, and central venous compression.

Renal compression to 15 mmHg results in a significant decrease in urine output, glomerular filtration rate (GFR), and effective renal blood flow (RBF) (32), which in turn can lead to an increase in renin release. Several studies have demonstrated an increase in renin secretion with intraabdominal insufflation (33–36) that returns to baseline levels with decompression of the abdomen (37). This increase in renin secretion is not seen with lower intraabdominal pressures (IAP) (34) and is thought to be due to redistribution of RBF from the outer cortex to the juxtamedullary zone (38–40). The failure of an angiotensin-converting enzyme inhibitor to prevent oliguria during laparoscopy does not support this theory (37).

Changes in renal arterial blood flow (RABF) and renal vein blood flow (RVBF) are also seen with changes in intraabdominal pressure. During pneumoperitoneum, the intraabdominal pressure is twice the vena caval pressure (41). It is not surprising that one study showed decreased urinary output at IAP greater than 15 mmHg that paralleled a decrease in RVBF (42). Although RABF is not affected at IAP below 10 mmHg, at levels above 20 mmHg, there is a 15% decrease in RABF, a 60% decrease in cortical perfusion, a 64% decrease in GFR, and a 50% decrease in urine output (43,44). Similar changes with central venous compression are also observed. With insufflation pressures at 10 mmHg, IVC flow decreases by 93% and aortic flow by 45% (45), both of which might have significant effects on renal plasma flow, GFR, and urine output.

Changes in urinary electrolytes (increased urinary potassium excretion and decreased urinary sodium excretion) during laparoscopy may be due to an elevation in serum aldosterone (46). In an experimental model, intravascular volume expansion during periods of increased intraabdominal pressure increased urine output and decreased renin and aldosterone levels (36).

Endothelin has also demonstrated its possible role with a 55% increase in the renal vein during pneumoperitoneum in the canine model (47). Furthermore, the use of endothelin receptor antagonists in the rat model during pneumoperitoneum resulted in less of a decrease in GFR (48).

CO_2 insufflation also increases antidiuretic hormone (ADH) concentrations (49,50). While ADH levels increased in 50% of women undergoing diagnostic laparoscopy (51), others have demonstrated no significant increase in ADH levels following insufflation of 15 mmHg (37). Some believe that the delay in desufflation diuresis may be linked to changes in ADH levels (52).

As mentioned previously, when encountering patients with underlying cardiac disease, renal disease, pulmonary disease, and diabetes mellitus and other comorbidities that may increase the magnitude of oliguria, careful intraoperative fluid management is important. Although attempting to maintain good urine output during the case is desirable, care should be taken with patients with compromised renal or cardiac function and consideration to invasive Swan–Ganz monitoring should be given. While it is a common belief that pneumoperitoneum of 25 mmHg is unsafe (53), the "gray zone" is in the 12–16 mmHg range. It is therefore recommended that insufflation pressures of 10–12 mmHg be employed, if possible, to prevent oliguria during gaseous laparoscopy (42,54), or less than 15 mmHg to minimize pulmonary complications. This usually allows good visualization with minimal and reversible hemodynamic stability and a decreased likelihood of other complications such as gas embolism and acid–base imbalances.

In conclusion, anesthetic considerations during laparoscopic surgery are very important and one should understand the predictable changes that may occur with insufflation. Knowledge of the effects of pneumoperitoneum and carbon dioxide, alterations in renal physiology, changes to the circulatory system, and the ability to quickly recognize and address

complications encountered with laparoscopy are paramount to
the proper care of these patients.

KEY POINTS

- Elevated CO_2 levels rarely cause cardiopulmonary
  complications.
- CO_2 diffusion is greater during extraperitoneal than
  intraperitoneal insufflation.
- Risks associated with hypercapnea are reduced by
  keeping pressures below 15 mmHg, avoiding subcutaneous emphysema and reducing procedure times.
- If gas embolism is suspected, terminate the procedure, release the pneumoperitoneum, increase the
  ventilated oxygen and place the patient in the left
  lateral decubitus position. Aspiration using a central
  venous catheter may be required.
- Renal function is altered during laparoscopy due to
  decreased cardiac output, renovascular compression,
  and central venous compression. The oliguria is
  usually transient and without long-term sequela.

REFERENCES

1. Pearce DJ. Respiratory acidosis and subcutaneous emphysema
   during laparoscopic cholecystectomy. Can J Anaesth 1994;
   41:314–316.

2. Rittenmeyer H. Carbon dioxide toxicity related to a laparoscopic procedure. J Post Anesth Care 1994; 9:157–161.

3. Wahba RWM, Mamazza J. Ventilatory requirements during
   laparoscopic cholecystectomy. Can J Anaesth 1993; 40:206–210.

4. Lee CM. Acute hypotension during laparoscopy: a case report.
   Anesth Analg 1975; 54:142–143.

5. Johannsen G, Andersen M, Juhl B. The effect of general
   anesthesia on the haemodynamic events during laparoscopy
   with CO2 insufflation. Acta Anaesth Scand 1989; 33:132–136.

6. Ekman LG, Abrahamsson J, Biber B, Forssman L, Milsom I, Sjoqvist BA. Hemodynamic changes during laparoscopy with positive end-expiratory pressure ventilation. Acta Anaesth Scand 1988; 32(6):447–453.

7. Iwase K, Takenaka H, Yagura A, Ishizaka T, Ohata T, Takagaki M, Oshima S. Hemodynamic changes during laparoscopic cholecystectomy in patients with heart disease. Endoscopy 1992; 24(9):771–773.

8. Graham AJ, Jirsch DW, Barrington KJ, Hayashi AH. Effects of intraabdominal CO2 insufflation in the piglet. J Pediatr Surg 1994; 29(9):1276–1280.

9. Hodgson C, McClelland RMA, Newton JR. Some effects of the peritoneal insufflation of carbon dioxide at laparoscopy. Anaesthesia 1970; 25:382.

10. Pillalamarri ED, Bhangdia P, Rudin RS, Chadhry RM, Tadoori PR, Abadir AR. Effect of CO2 pneumoperitoneum during laparoscopy on ABG's, end-tidal CO2, and cardiovascular dynamics. Anesthesiology 1983; 59:A424.

11. Magno R, Medegard A, Bengtsson R, Tronstad SE. Acid–base balance during laparoscopy. The effects of intraperitoneal insufflation of carbon dioxide on acid–base balance during controlled ventilation. Acta Obstet Gynecol Scand 1979; 58:81.

12. Bongard FS, Pianim NA, Leighton TA, Dubecz S, Davis IP, Lippmann M, Klein S, Liu SY. Helium insufflation for laparoscopic operation. Surg Gynecol Obstet 1993; 177:140.

13. Neuberger TJ, Andrus CH, Wittgen CM, Wade TP, Kaminski DL. Prospective comparison of helium versus carbon dioxide pneumoperitoneum. Gastrointest Endosc 1994; 40:30.

14. Wolf JS, Monk TG, McDougall EM, McLennan BL, Clayman RV. The extraperitoneal approach and subcutaneous emphysema are associated with greater absorption of carbon dioxide during laparoscopic renal surgery. J Urol 1995; 154:959–963.

15. Smith I, Benzie RJ, Gordon NLM, Kelman GR, Swapp GH. Cardiovascular effects of peritoneal insufflation of carbon dioxide for laparoscopy. Br Med J 1971; 3(771):410–411.

16. Motew M, Ivankovich AD, Bieniarz J, Albrecht RF, Zahed B, Scommegna A. Cardiovascular effects of acid–base and blood

gas changes during laparoscopy. Am J Obstet Gynecol 1973; 115:1002.

17. Wakizaka Y, Sano S, Koike Y, Nakanishi Y, Uchino J. Changes of arterial CO2 (PaCO2) and urine output by carbon dioxide insufflation of the peritoneal cavity during laparoscopic cholecystectomy. J Jap Surg Soc 1994; 95:336.

18. Kent RB III. Subcutaneous emphysema and hypercarbia following laparoscopic cholecystectomy. Arch Surg 1991; 126: 1154.

19. Sosa RE, Weingram J, Stein B, Lyons JM, Poppas D, Bander NH, Vaughn ED Jr. Hypercarbia in laparoscopic pelvic lymph node dissection. J Urol 1992; 147:246.

20. Hall D, Goldstein A, Tynan E, Braunstein L. Profound hypercarbia late in the course of laparoscopic cholecystectomy: detection by continuous capnometry. Anesthesiology 1993; 79: 173.

21. Mullett CE, Viale JP, Sagnard PE, Miellet CC, Ruynat LG, Counioux HC, Motin JP, Boulez JP, Dargent DM, Annat GJ. Pulmonary CO_2 elimination during surgical procedures using intra- or extraperitoneal CO_2 insufflation. Anesth Analg 1993; 76:622.

22. Wolf JS, Jr, Carrier S, Stoller ML. Intraperitoneal versus extraperitoneal insufflation of carbon dioxide as for laparoscopy. J Endourol 1995; 9:63.

23. Adams JB, Moore RG, Micali S, Marco AP, Kavoussi LR. Laparoscopic genitourinary surgery utilizing 20 mm Hg intra-abdominal pressure. J Laparoendosc Adv Surg Tech A 1999; 9(2):131–134.

24. Blaser A, Rosset P. Fatal carbon dioxide embolism as an unreported complication of retroperitoneoscopy. Surg Endosc 1999; 13(7):713–714.

25. O'Sullivan DC, Micali S, Averch TD, Buffer S, Reyerson T, Schulam P, Kavoussi LR. Factors involved in gas embolism after laparoscopic injury to inferior vena cava. J Endourol 1998; 12(2):149–154.

26. Fahy BG, Hasnain JU, Flowers JL, Plotkin JS, Odonkor P, Ferguson MK. Transesophageal echocardiographic detection

of gas embolism and cardiac valvular dysfunction during laparoscopic nephrectomy. Anesth Analg 1999; 88(3):500–504.

27. Diakun TA. Carbon dioxide embolism: successful resuscitation with cardiopulmonary bypass. Anesthesiology 1991; 74:1151–1153.

28. Behnia R, Holley HS, Milad M. Successful early intervention in air embolism during hysteroscopy. J Clin Anesth 1997; 9(3):248–250.

29. McAllister JD, D'Altorio RA, Snyder A. CT findings after uncomplicated percutaneous laparoscopic cholecystectomy. J Comp Assist Tomog 1991; 15:770–772.

30. Philips JM. Complications in laparoscopy. Int J Gynecol Obstet 1977; 95:157–162.

31. Rudston-Brown BC, MacLennan D, Warriner CB, Phang PT. Effect of subcutaneous carbon dioxide insufflation on arterial pCO_2. Am J Surg 1996; 171(5):460–463.

32. Razvi HA, Fields D, Vargas JC, Vaughan ED Jr, Vukasin A, Sosa RE. Oliguria during laparoscopic surgery: evidence for direct renal parenchymal compression as an etiologic factor. J Endourol 1996; 10(1):1–4.

33. O'Leary E, Hubbard K, Tormey W, Cunningham AJ. Laparoscopic cholecystectomy after pneumoperitoneum and changes in position. Br J Anaesth 1996; 76(5):640–644.

34. Koivusalo AM, Kellokumpu I, Scheinin M, Tikkanen I, Halme L, Lindgren L. Randomized comparison of the neuroendocrine response to laparoscopic cholecystectomy using either conventional or abdominal wall lift techniques. Br J Surg 1996; 83(11):1532–1536.

35. Diebel LN, Wilson RF, Dulchavsky SA, Saxe J. Effects of increased intraabdominal pressure on hepatic arterial, portal venous, and hepatic microcirculatory blood flow. J Trauma 1992; 33(2):279–283.

36. Bloomfield GL, Blocher CR, Fakhry IF, Sica DA, Sugerman HJ. Elevated intra-abdominal pressure increases plasma renin activity and aldosterone levels. J Trauma 1997; 42(6):997–1004.

37. Vukasin A, Shichman S, Hom D, et al. The mechanism of oliguria associated with intra-abdominal insufflation. Annual AUA Meeting, 1995.

38. Kishimoto T, Maedawa M, Abe Y, Yamamoto K. Intrarenal distribution of blood flow and renin release during renal venous pressure elevation. Kidney Int 1973; 4(4):259–266.

39. Abe Y, Kishimoto T, Yamamoto K, Ueda J. Intrarenal distribution of blood flow during ureteral and venous pressure elevation. Am J Physiol 1973; 224(4):746–751.

40. Miyazaki M, McNay J. Redistribution of renal cortical blood flow during ureteral occlusion and renal venous constriction. Proc Soc Exp Biol Med 1971; 138(2):454–461.

41. Chiu AW, Chang LS, Birkett DH, Babayan RK. The impact of pneumoperitoneum, pneumoretroperitoneum, and gasless laparoscopy on the systemic and renal hemodynamics. J Am Coll Surg 1995; 181(5):397–406.

42. McDougall EM, Monk TG, Wolf JS Jr, Hicks M, Clayman RV, Gardner S, Humphrey PA, Sharp T, Martin K. The effect of prolonged pneumoperitoneum on renal function in an animal model. J Am Coll Surg 1996; 182(4):317–328.

43. Chiu AW, Azadzoi KM, Hatzichristou DG, Siroky MB, Krane RJ, Babayan RK. Effects of intra-abdominal pressure on renal tissue perfusion during laparoscopy. J Endourol 1994; 8(2): 99–103.

44. Cisek LJ, Peters CA. Pneumoperitoneum is associated with acute but not chronic alteration of renal function. J Endourol 1997; 11:54.

45. Kirsch AJ, Hensle TW, Chang DT, Kayton ML, Olsson CA, Sawczuk IS. Renal effects of CO_2 insufflation: oliguria and acute renal dysfunction in a rat pneumoperitoneum model. Urology 1994; 43(4):453–459.

46. Chiu AW, Chang LS, Birkett DH, Babayan RK. Changes in urinary output and electrolytes during gaseous and gasless laparoscopy. Urol Res 1996; 24(6):361–366.

47. Hamilton BD, Chow GK, Stowe NT, et al. The effect of renal vein compression on renal function: a canine model for laparoscopic surgery. J Endourol 1997; 11:53.

48. Stowe NT, Sung GT, Sobel JJ, et al. Endothelin antagonist attenuation pneumoperitoneum-induced fall in GFR in a rat model. J Endourol 1998; 12(1):97.

49. Le Roith D, Bark H, Nyska M, Glick SM. The effect of abdominal pressure on plasma antidiuretic hormone levels in the dog. J Surg Res 1982; 32(1):65–69.

50. Ortega A, Peters J, Incarbone R, Estrada L, Ehsan A, Kwan Y, Spencer CJ, Moore-Jeffries E, Kuchta K, Nicoloff JT. A prospective randomized comparison of the metabolic and stress hormonal responses of laparoscopic and open cholecystectomy. J Am Coll Surg 1996; 183(3):249–256.

51. Viinamaki O, Punnonen R. Vasopressin release during laparoscopy: role of increased intra-abdominal pressure. Lancet 1982; 1(8264):175–176.

52. Seiba M, Schulsinger D, Sosa RE. The renal physiology of laparoscopic surgery. AUA Update Ser 2000; XIX(23):180.

53. Williams M, Simms H. Abdominal compartment syndrome: case reports and implications for management in critically ill patients. Am Surg 1997; 63(6):555–558.

54. Richards WO, Scovill W, Shin B, Reed W. Acute renal failure associated with increased intra-abdominal pressure. Ann Surg 1983; 197(2):183–187.

2

Complications of Laparoscopic Access

MATTHEW T. GETTMAN

Department of Urology, Mayo Clinic,
Rochester, Minnesota, U.S.A.

INTRODUCTION

Abdominal access is fundamental for all laparoscopic procedures; however, a variety of complications are associated with
placement of trocars, the Veress needle, or the Hasson cannula. In recent investigations, the incidence of access complications for laparoscopic procedures in gynecology and general
surgery is 0.18–1.4% (1–6). Despite the rarity of injuries,
access complications occur in greater frequency than other
complications associated with laparoscopic cholecystectomy
and common gynecologic procedures (4,5,7). In reports published between 1993 and 1996, the incidence of access complications associated with urologic procedures was 1.8–5.4%

(8–12). For reports published between 1999 and 2001, the incidence of access complications was 0.4–2.0% (13–16). Despite the decreasing incidence of access complications, all urologists should be aware of the possible injuries and their management.

While many access complications are associated with minimal morbidity, others are life-threatening, mandate an immediate open conversion, or require subsequent operative interventions (17–19). Using insurance claims information and data from United States Food and Drug Administration (FDA), Chandler and colleagues (19) reviewed 594 access complications occurring in 509 patients between 1980 and 1999. Injury severity included temporary major impairment, long-term major impairment, and death in 55%, 22%, and 13% of patients, respectively (19). Access complications occur intraoperatively when access equipment is malpositioned. As a consequence, all intraabdominal organs are at risk when entering the abdomen. The postoperative development of site complications also represents an adverse consequence of laparoscopic access. In addition, some postoperative complications are a delayed manifestation of occult intraoperative injuries. Regardless the cause, prompt identification and management decreases the morbidity and significance of entry complications (6,19).

Despite the introduction of access equipment with proposed safety features and the touted benefits of one access technique over another, advantages of a specific access technique have not been proven in appropriately constructed scientific trials (1,5,19,20). In reality, access complications are likely influenced by many factors including surgical experience and technique, familiarity with the access equipment, and unique patient-related issues (13). Optimizing as many of these factors as possible may provide the best prevention of access injuries (1,21). This chapter summarizes the recognition, evaluation, management, and prevention of intraoperative and postoperative complications related to abdominal access. Issues regarding injury to organs or vascular structures, hernia, and tumor seeding of port sites are covered in other chapters of this book.

PREVENTION STRATEGIES

Preoperative Evaluation

Patients at high risk for access complications are identified during the preoperative evaluation (8,21). For all patients, the past surgical history is reviewed and the location of abdominal scars is noted on physical examination. Postoperative adhesions increase the risk of access-related bowel injury. Brill and associates reported that the incidence of intestinal adhesions associated with a previous midline or Pfannenstiel incision was 57% and 27%, respectively. Of the 360 patients included in the report, access-related bowel or omental injuries were observed in 6% (21 patients) (22). Lecuru and colleagues (23) similarly noted that access complications were significantly higher for patients after laparotomy than those without prior abdominal surgery. Secondary to abdominal wall laxity and the possibility of bowel adhesions, women are at risk for access injuries following pregnancy. Obesity is another risk factor for entry complications (24,25). Mendoza and coworkers (25) noted a 22% complication rate among 125 markedly obese patients undergoing urologic laparoscopy. Technical difficulties including poor transillumination of the abdominal wall and difficult trocar insertion were observed in 61% and 14% of patients, respectively (25). On the other hand, children and extremely thin adults are also at risk for access complications because of decreased muscle mass and proximity of the great vessels to the abdominal wall (24). In addition, the presence of physical deformity (spine abnormalities, body contractures) predisposes these patients to access complications (26,27). Finally, an awareness of adverse medical factors, such as hepatomegaly, can reduce the risk of access injury.

Patient Preparation

All adults should have a urinary catheter and oral-gastric tube placed preoperatively to minimize the risk of bladder or bowel injuries (8,21). At a minimum, one large-bore intravenous line is placed preoperatively (21). A type and screen is

performed for two units of packed red blood cells and prophy-
lactic antibiotics are administered (13,21). Because of the risk
of bowel distention, nitrous oxide is avoided during laparoscopic procedures (28). Some investigators have additionally
recommended a preoperative bowel prep to decompress the
bowel, increase the working area of the peritoneum, and minimize the morbidity of access-related bowel injuries (13,29).

Equipment

Disposable equipment and nondisposable equipment are
available for laparoscopic access (30,31). The proper function
of all equipment (disposable and nondisposable) is verified
before attempting to enter the abdomen (16,30). To minimize
the risk of access injuries with nondisposable equipment, the
cutting mechanism should be resharpened about every 20
cases. A sharp tip facilitates instrument insertion with less
force and more control (32). Disposable trocars often incorpo-
rate a safety shield feature designed to prevent access complications. Safety shields are spring-loaded plastic coverings
that advance in front of the trocar blade when resistance to
cutting is not detected (18,30). To date, safety shields have
not eliminated access complications (24,33). In an assessment
of Medical Device Reports from the FDA between 1993 and
1996, Bhoyrul et al. (18) found 28 fatal injuries associated
with safety-shielded trocars as well as 355 nonfatal vascular
injuries and 116 bowel injuries. In addition, the FDA has
not recognized safety shields as a bona fide way to minimize
access complications (18,19).

New trocar designs have been introduced with a goal of
increasing access safety. Expandable access systems permit
stabilization of the abdominal wall during placement of
sheaths that convert the forces of entry from axial to radial
(19,34). Expandable devices have been used in the adult and
pediatric population as well as in patients with prior abdominal surgery (19). The expanding devices obviate the need for
fascial closure in many cases and may decrease the risk of
abdominal wall blood vessel injury. Unfortunately, injuries
related to blind Veress needle placement are reported with

this access system. In the report by Shekarriz and colleagues (35), Veress needle liver punctures occurred in 9% of patients. Routine subcostal placement of the Veress needle, however, may have contributed to the reported incidence of solid organ injuries. A trocar-less rotational access cannula (TRAC) was also recently developed for abdominal entry (36). The reusable threaded cannula is rotated into position under endoscopic vision thereby limiting axial forces of entry. Similar to the expandable trocar devices, fascial closure is often not required. In a prospective clinical trial by Termanian (37), 203 unselected females underwent gynecologic laparoscopy without access complications.

Surgical Approach

The position of planned trocar incisions and the method of abdominal entry are frequently influenced by physical findings. Initial access is commonly performed at the umbilicus using either an open or closed technique. Open access involves trocar placement under direct vision, whereas the closed access refers to blind trocar placement. For patients with a history of abdominal surgery, primary access is usually obtained as far as possible from surgical scars (31,38). Secondary trocars are then placed under direct vision. For patients with prior abdominal surgery, the left upper quadrant has alternatively been used as a site for initial access (39). When extensive surgical scars are present across the entire abdomen, retroperitoneoscopy is another treatment option (16,38,40). In fact, Fahlenkamp and associates (16) reported that the risk of visceral injuries was three-fold higher for a transperitoneal vs. a retroperitoneal laparoscopic approach. After placing all trocars, the intraabdominal contents and trocar sites (primary and secondary) are inspected for access injury. In some cases, access injuries can involve multiple organ systems (19). Visual inspection is especially important whenever access inadvertently occurs in an uncontrolled manner. The laparoscope, a laparoscopic suction/irrigator, and a laparotomy set (including vascular clamps) should be readily available during access (21).

Closed access remains widely practiced because it is less expensive, easier to perform, and require less operative time than traditional open access (6,9,16). During closed access, pneumoperitoneum is most commonly established with the Veress needle (Table 1) followed by blind placement of the primary trocar (Table 2) (16,31). Pneumoperitoneum, however, does not prevent injuries associated with blind trocar placement. Furthermore, blind Veress needle placement is also associated with significant complicat ions (2,17). Some investigators therefore advocate direct trocar insertion without pneumoperitoneum. Unfortunately, results of this closed access method are also conflicting (1,6,17,20,41).

Open access is traditionally performed by inserting a Hasson cannula through a mini-laparotomy incision (Table 3). Open trocar placement was developed, in part, to decrease the risk of bowel and vascular injuries during access (42). Among 5284 laparoscopic procedures, Hasson reported a 0.5% overall complications rate (27 patients). The most common complication was a wound infection (21 patients), while only one patient had a bowel injury and none had vascular injuries (43). Because of technical limitations (longer time requirement to perform, more difficult to perform in some patients, problems maintaining pneumoperitoneum), open access was not immediately embraced. Nonetheless, open access has routinely been recommended for children, pregnant females, obese patients, extremely thin patients, and select patients with prior abdominal surgery (11,12,17). Furthermore, based on complications noted with closed access, open access is increasingly performed as the first-line method for abdominal entry (1,2,6,44).

With increased utilization of the open access, major complications (including bowel and vascular injuries) have also been reported with these techniques (19,44–47). Hanney and colleagues (47) reported two aortic injuries associated with open access. The first injury (related to surgical technique) occurred with a thin female, whereas the second injury was attributed to a faulty reusable Hasson cannula. Furthermore, Chandler and colleagues (19) reported 18 access complications

Table 1 Veress Needle Placement

A. Patient is rotated on the operating room table into a relatively horizontal position

B. Intended position of Veress needle is as far as possible from surgical scars

C. Abdominal wall is stabilized with towel clips

D. Veress needle is placed slowly through small stab incision

E. Veress needle is inserted at slight angle towards pelvis. Excessive force should never be required

F. Resistance is met as needle traverses the abdominal fascia and the peritoneum

G. Confirmatory tests are performed to assess position of the Veress needle

   1. Aspiration test: If needle correctly positioned, attempts to aspirate needle are unsuccessful. Character and color of aspirated fluid provide clues to access injury

   2. Drop test: Drop of saline placed at hub of needle. If the needle is correctly positioned, saline drops quickly into the peritoneal cavity and not aspirated

   3. Saline injection test: Saline (5–10 cm^3) injected through the needle. If the needle is correctly positioned, attempts to aspirate saline are unsuccessful

   4. Insufflation test: Attach needle to insufflator at low CO_2 flow settings. If intraabdominal pressures 4–8 mmHg, correct position of needle is suggested. Pressures >8 mmHg suggest incorrect position or needle contact with intraabdominal structure

H. Insufflate at high CO_2 flow settings only when satisfied with intraabdominal needle position (Air embolus or preperitoneal insufflation can occur if CO_2 instilled before confirming intraabdominal position of needle.)

I. Place primary trocar only after sufficient pneumoperitoneum is attained

Table 2 Trocar Placement

A. Operating room table is positioned at comfortable height that allows surgeon's shoulders to be slightly abducted

B. Insertion away from previous surgical scars (primary trocar) or visualized adhesions (secondary trocar). Abdominal wall is transilluminated before secondary trocar placement to avoid injury to abdominal wall blood vessels

C. Adequate skin incision to allow the trocar and obturator to pass freely through the abdominal wall

D. Subcutaneous tissues divided to the level of fascia

E. Abdominal wall stabilized with towel clips

F. Trocar placed with two hands using minimal force and slow twisting motion of the entire upper extremity. Excessive force should never be required

---

(causing three deaths) related to Hasson cannula. In the report, major vascular and bowel injuries accounted for 67% of the complications. In a survey of 18 gynecologists that switched from the closed to the open access technique, Penfield (48) reported that bowel injuries and wound infections were the most common complications. In a comparison of open

Table 3 Hasson Cannula Placement

A. Patient is rotated on the operating room table into a relatively horizontal position

B. Incision is performed (10–12 mm in length) and sub-cutaneous tissues divided to identify fascia

C. Fascia is secured on either side of planned incision and fascia is sharply incised

D. Peritoneum is identified, grasp, and sharply divided

E. Intraabdominal position confirmed with finger palpation

F. Cannula inserted under direct visualization

G. Cannula secured to prevent loss of CO_2 pneumoperitoneum

---

and closed access during laparoscopic cholecystectomy, Wherry and colleagues (44) noted that more injuries were related to the use of the Hasson cannula ($n = 11$) than the Veress needle ($n = 4$). On the other hand, open access is associated with a lower complication rate than closed access in other investigations (1,17,33).

Open access can also be performed with a visual obturator. Visual obturators are handled insertion devices that permit conventional trocar placement under direct laparoscopic vision (17,49). The Visiport (US Surgical, Norwalk, CT) allows for stepwise trocar placement with a triggered cutting mechanism, while the Optiview (Ethicon Surgical, Cincinnati, OH) is placed with a twisting motion under direct vision (17,50). Similar to open access performed with the Hasson cannula, visual obturators permit primary trocar placement under direct vision (17,49). In contrast to the Hasson technique, optical trocars requires less insertion time and minimizes CO_2 leakage. Marcovich and associates (50) evaluated efficacy of the Optiview device as the initial method of access ($n = 4$) or when initial access could not be obtained with the Veress needle ($n = 22$). Overall, Optiview access was obtained in 96% of cases and no complications were recorded. Similarly, String and coworkers (49) successfully used the Optiview for open access in 650 patients with a complication rate of 0.3%. However, the risks of access with optical trocars are evolving. In a recent Medical Device Report by the FDA, both major vascular and visceral injuries were associated with optical trocar devices (17,18).

At the end of the laparoscopic procedure, trocar sites and the abdomen are again inspected for occult injury (24). Careful closure of the surgical incisions is imperative since most postoperative access complications are in some way or other related to the trocar site (33). For example, Mayol and colleagues (33) reported that 95% of access complications were related to wound infections, trocar hernias, or abdominal wall hematomas. To minimize the risk of postoperative complications, all fascial defects in children and fascial defects >5 mm mm in adults are closed (13). Fascial closure can be cumbersome with standard surgical instruments. Alternatively, a fascial closure device can be used for trocar site closure under laparoscopic monitoring (Fig. 1) (51).

Surgical experience and careful surgical technique are very important factors in the prevention of access injuries (11,16,20,24,27,48,52,53). Dixon and Carillo (53) evaluated seven major vascular injuries that occurred in five patients during elective laparoscopic procedures. The operating sur-

(A)

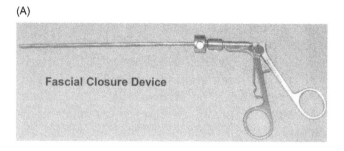

(B)

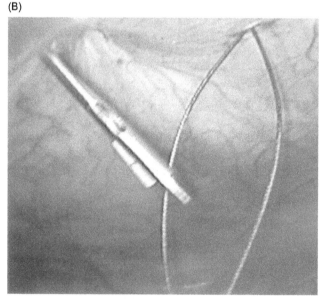

Figure 1 (A) Fascial closure device (Storz endoscopy) permits closure of trocar sites under direct laparoscopic visualization. (B) After the suture is introduced lateral to fascial defect, the empty device is reintroduced on the opposite side to grasp the suture and finish the closure.

geon for these five patients had previously performed <10, 15, 20, <5, and 15 laparoscopic cases, respectively. Likewise, Hashizume and colleagues (2) noted that the incidence of access complications decreased yearly as increased surgical experience was gained in laparoscopy. In stepwise logistic analysis performed by Jansen and coworkers (3), the development of laparoscopic complications (access and nonaccess) requiring laparotomy was predicted by surgical experience and a history of prior laparotomy. Furthermore, Cadeddu and colleagues (14) recently reported that advanced training favorably impacts the incidence of complications (access and nonaccess) in urologic laparoscopy. For surgeons completing at least 12 months of concentrated laparoscopic training, the incidence of complications in the initial 20, 30, and 40 cases was identical.

INTRAOPERATIVE COMPLICATIONS

Air Embolus

An air embolus is a rare, life-threatening complication that can occur during laparoscopic access (21,28,54). Prompt recognition and management are required for a favorable outcome. An air embolus develops when CO_2 is inadvertently introduced into the blood stream (21,54). This complication most commonly occurs during access when the Veress needle is accidentally placed into the vena cava or iliac vein and instilled CO_2 is embolized to the right heart (28,54,55). Less commonly, an air embolus can develop in conjunction with a trocar injury. In either case, an air embolus is usually manifested during the first few minutes of the laparoscopic procedure (28).

Embolized CO_2 creates an "air lock" in the right heart that impedes blood flow into the pulmonary circulation (21). The "air lock" decreases the blood flow through the pulmonary vein with subsequent left ventricular failure and immediate vascular collapse. An air embolus is accompanied by a pronounced decrease in end-tidal CO_2, a dramatic decrease in oxygen saturation, and profound hypotension (54,55). A widening of the QRS complex, tachydysrhythmias, or development of a right heart strain pattern can also occur on the electrocardiogram (28,55). Classically, a mill-wheel murmur is heard during chest auscultation. If an air embolus is suspected, the insufflator is immediately turned off and all laparoscopic ports opened for escape of CO_2. Furthermore, the patient is immediately placed in a steep Trendelenburg, left lateral decubitus position (left side down, right side up) to minimize the effect of the right ventricular "air lock" (21). General resuscitative maneuvers are then started as well as attempts to aspirate CO_2 from the right heart via a central venous catheter (21). As soon as possible, a laparotomy is performed to repair the underlying vascular injury.

Preperitoneal Insufflation

Preperitoneal is a relatively minor complication that occurs when CO_2 is instilled proximal to the peritoneal cavity (21,25). Preperitoneal insufflation makes peritoneal access more difficult because the CO_2 decreases abdominal compliance, increases the distance from the skin to the peritoneum, and reduces the working volume of the peritoneal cavity (12,21). Abdominal asymmetry during CO_2 instillation suggests preperitoneal insufflation. High insufflation pressures (>10 mmHg) and a low instilled CO_2 volume (<1 L) often accompany the physical findings (31). In some instances, preperitoneal insufflation is not recognized until the primary trocar is positioned. If preperitoneal insufflation occurs, CO_2 is evacuated as possible from the preperitoneal space and access is performed at a new site. If a large volume of CO_2 was instilled into the preperitoneal space, open access may be preferable (21).

POSTOPERATIVE COMPLICATIONS

Wound Infection

Wound infections are a relatively common minor complications of laparoscopy (43,48). Local tissue trauma and inflammation of the trocar site contribute to the development of a wound infection. Typical signs and symptoms of cellulitis accompany trocar site infections. Most infections respond rapidly with antibiotics. In the case of purulent drainage, wound debridement is performed. In most cases, wound infections have minimal impact, but necrotizing fascitis has developed at a trocar site after laparoscopy (56). In addition, Hurd and colleagues (57) have reported abscess development at a trocar site that was effectively managed with surgical drainage, irrigation, and antibiotics. In addition, wound infections have also been reported as a risk factor for trocar site hernias (33).

Abdominal Wall Hematoma

Unrecognized or incompletely controlled injuries of abdominal wall vessels can contribute to the formation of abdominal wall hematomas (57). In fact, Mayol and colleagues (33) reported that abdominal wall hematomas were the most access complication among 403 patients undergoing laparoscopy. Bulging, erythema, bruising, or abdominal wall asymmetry near the trocar site are clues to the presence of an abdominal wall hematoma (8). The size of the hematoma often determines the degree of discomfort, as small hematomas typically have little associated pain. Other patients have lateralizing abdominal wall pain with signs and symptoms of significant hemorrhage (5). Many abdominal wall hematomas resolve spontaneously without additional intervention (33). For patients with ongoing hemorrhage or hematoma expansion, surgical exploration is required to evacuate the hematoma and control the bleeding (33,57,58).

CONCLUSION

A variety of intraoperative and postoperative complications can occur during laparoscopic access; however, the incidence of access complications in urology is very low and appears to be decreasing. Access complications are influenced by many factors including surgical experience and technique, familiarity of laparoscopic equipment, and patient-related factors. Despite the introduction of technologic modifications to increase the safety of abdominal entry, all access equipment is associated with complications and no method of access is superior. While some access complications are life-threatening or require immediate open conversion, many injuries have limited impact on the patient or the ability to perform the planned surgical intervention using minimally invasive techniques.

Access complications are minimized by a careful preoperative evaluation, thorough patient preparation, and excellent surgical technique. A low index of suspicion for entry-related injuries can decrease the impact and significance of these complications both intraoperatively and postoperatively. When faced with an access complication, a stepwise approach should be taken to fully evaluate the problem, exclude the possibility of concurrent access injuries, and devise a treatment plan that minimizes morbidity associated with the injury and maximizes safety for the patient.

REFERENCES

1. Catarci M, Carlini M, Gentileschi P, Santoro E. Lap Group Roma. Major and minor injuries during the creation of pneumoperitoneum: a multicenter study of 12, cases. Surg Endosc 2001; 15:566–569.

2. Hashizume M, Sugimachi K. Study Group of Endoscopic Surgery in Kyushu, Japan. Needle and trocar injury during laparoscopic surgery. Surg Endosc 1997; 11:1198–1201.

3. Jansen FW, Kapiteyn K, Trimbos-Kemper T, Hermans J, Trimbos JB. Complications of laparoscopy: a prospective multicentre observational study. Br J Obstet Gynaecol 1997; 104:595–600.

4. Ahmad SA, Schuricht AL, Azurin DJ, Arroyo LR, Paskin DL, Bar AH, Kirkland ML. Complications of laparoscopic cholecystectomy: the experience of a university-affiliated teaching hospital. J Laparoendosc Adv Tech A 1997; 7:29–35.

5. Bateman BG, Kolp LA, Hoeger K. Complications of laparoscopy-operative and diagnostic. Fert Steril 1996; 66:30–35.

6. Schafer M, Lauper M, Krahenbuhl L. Trocar and Veress needle injuries during laparoscopy. Surg Endosc 2001; 15:275–289.

7. Leonard F, Lecuru F, Rizk E, Chasset S, Robin F, Taurelle R. Perioperative morbidity of gynecological laparoscopy: a prospective monocenter observational study. Acta Obstet Gynecol Scand 2000; 79:129–134.

8. Kavoussi LR, Sosa E, Chandhoke P, Chodak G, Clayman RV, Hadley HR, Loughlin KR, Ruckle HC, Rukstalis D, Schuessler W, Segura J, Vancaille T, Winfield HN. Complications of laparoscopic pelvic lymph node dissection. J Urol 1993; 149: 322–325.

9. Thomas R, Steele R, Ahuja S. Complications of urological laparoscopy: a standardized 1 institution experience. J Urol 1996; 156:469–471.

10. Gill IS, Kavoussi LR, Clayman RV, Ehrlich R, Evans R, Fuchs G, Gersham A, Hulbert JC, McDougall EM, Rosenthal T, Schuessler WW, Shepard T. Complications of laparoscopic nephrectomy in 185 patients: multi-institutional review. J Urol 1995; 154:479–483.

11. Peters CA. Complications in pediatric urologic laparoscopy: results of a survey. J Urol 1996; 155:1070–1073.

12. Parra RO, Hagood PG, Boullier JA, Cummings JM, Mehan DJ. Complications of laparoscopic urological surgery: experience at St. Louis University. J Urol 1994; 151:681–684.

13. Soulie M, Seguin P, Richeux L, Mouly P, Vazzoler N, Pontonnier F, Plante P. Urological complications of laparoscopic surgery: experience with 350 procedures at a single center. J Urol 2001; 165:1960–1963.

14. Cadeddu JA, Wolfe JS Jr, Nakada S, Chen R, Shalhav A, Bishoff JT, Hamilton B, Schulam PG, Dunn M, Hoenig D, Fabrizo M, Hedican S, Averch TD. Complications of laparoscopic procedures after concentrated training in urological laparoscopy. J Urol 2001; 168:2109–2111.

15. Soulie M, Salomon L, Seguin P, Mervant C, Mouly P, Hoznek A, Antiphon P, Plante P, Abbou CC. Multi-institutional study of complications in 1085 laparoscopic urologic procedures. Urology 2001; 58:899–903.

16. Fahlenkamp D, Rassweiler J, Forana P, Frede T, Loening SA. Complications of laparoscopic procedures in urology: experi-

ence with 2407 procedures at 4 German centers. J Urol 1999; 162:765–771.

17. Philips PA, Amaral JF. Abdominal access complications in laparoscopic surgery. J Am Coll Surg 2001; 192:525–536.

18. Bhoyrul S, Vierra MA, Nezhat CR, Krummel TM, Way LW. Trocar injuries in laparoscopic surgery. J Am Coll Surg 2001; 192:677–683.

19. Chandler JG, Corson SL, Way LW. Three spectra of laparoscopic entry complications. J Am Coll Surg 2001; 192: 478–491.

20. Woolcott R. The safety of laparoscopy performed by direct trocar insertion and carbon dioxide insufflation under vision. Aust New Zealand J Obstet Gynecol 1997; 37:216–219.

21. See WA, Monk TG, Weldon BC. Complications of laparoscopy: strategies for prevention and treatment. In: Clayman RV, McDougall EM, eds. Laparoscopic Urology. St. Louis: Quality Medical Publishing, 1993:183–205.

22. Brill AI, Nezhat F, Nezhat CH, Nezhat C. The incidence of adhesions after prior laparotomy: a laparoscopic appraisal. Obstet Gynecol 1995; 85:269–272.

23. Lecuru F, Leonard F, Philippe JJ, Rizk E, Robin F, Taurelle R. Laparoscopy in patients with prior surgery: results of the blind approach. JSLS 2001; 5:13–16.

24. Chapron CM, Pierre F, Lacroix S, Querleu D, Lansac J, Dubuisson JB. Major vascular injuries during gynecologic laparoscopy. J Am Coll Surg 1997; 185:476–481.

25. Mendoza D, Newman RC, Albala D, Cohen MS, Tewari A, Lingeman J, Wong M, Kavoussi L, Adams J, Moore R, Winfield H, Glascock JM, Das S, Munch L, Grasso M, Dickinson M, Clayman R, Nakada S, McDougall EM, Wolf JS, Hulbert J, Leveilee RJ, Houshair A, Carson C. Laparoscopic complications in markedly obese urologic patients (a multi-institutional review). Urology 1996; 48:562–567.

26. Esposito C, Ascione G, Garipoli V, DeBernardo G, Esposito G. Complications of pediatric laparoscopic surgery. Surg Endosc 1997; 11:655–657.

27. Soderstrom RM. Injuries to major blood vessels during endoscopy. J Am Assoc Gynecol Laparosc 1997; 4:395–398.

28. Wolf JS Jr, Stoller ML. The physiology of laparoscopy: basic principles, complications, and other considerations. J Urol 1994; 152:294–302..

29. Clayman RV. Secondary trocar placement. In: Clayman RV, McDougall EM, eds. Laparoscopic Urology. St. Louis: Quality Medical Publishing, 1993:66–81.

30. Winfield HN. Abdominal access: initial trocar placement. In: Clayman RV, McDougall EM, eds. Laparoscopic Urology. St. Louis: Quality Medical Publishing, 1993:38–50.

31. Kavoussi LR. Establishing the pneumoperitoneum. In: Clayman RV, McDougall EM, eds. Laparoscopic Urology. St. Louis: Quality Medical Publishing, 1993:28–36.

32. Kelty CJ, Super PA, Stoddard CJ. The driving force in trocar insertion. Surg Endosc 2000; 14:1045–1046.

33. Mayol J, Garcia-Aguilar J, Ortiz-Oshiro E, De-Diego Carmona JA, Fernandez-Represa JA. Risks of the minimal access approach for laparoscopic surgery: multivariate analysis of morbidity related to umbilical trocar insertion. World J Surg 1997; 21:529–533.

34. Schulam PG, Hedican SP, Docimo SG. Radially expanding trocar system for open laparoscopic access. Urology 1999; 54:727–729.

35. Shekarriz B, Gholami SS, Rudnick DM, Duh QY, Stroller ML. Radially expanding laparoscopic access for renal/adrenal surgery. Urology 2001; 58:683–687.

36. Termanian AM. Laparoscopy without trocars. Surg Endosc 1997; 11:815–818.

37. Termanian AM. A trocarless, reusable, visual-access cannula for safer laparoscopy; an update. J Am Assoc Gynecol Laparosc 1998; 5:1434–1438.

38. Chen RN, Moore RG, Cadeddu JA, Schulam P, Hedican SP, Llorens SA, Kavoussi LR. Laparoscopic renal surgery in patients at high risk for intra-abdominal or retroperitoneal scarring. J Endourol 1998; 12:143–147.

39. Audebert AJM, Gomel V. Role of microlaparoscopy in the diagnosis of peritoneal and visceral adhesions and in the prevention of bowel injury associated with blind trocar insertion. Fert Steril 2000; 73:631–635.

40. Rassweiler JJ, Seeman O, Frede T, Henkel TO, Alken P. Retroperitonescopy: experience with 200 cases. J Urol 1998; 160:1265–1269.

41. Yerdel MA, Karayalcin K, Koyuncu A, Akin B, Koysoy C, Turkcapar AG, Erverdi N, Alacayir I, Bumin C, Aras N. Direct trocar insertion versus Veress needle insertion in laparoscopic cholecystectomy. Am J Surg 1999; 177:247–249.

42. Hasson HM. A modified instrument and method for laparoscopy. Am J Obstet Gynecol 1971; 110:886–887.

43. Hasson HM, Rotman C, Rana N, Kumari NA. Open laparoscopy: 29-year experience. Obstet Gynecol 2000; 96:763–766.

44. Wherry DC, Marohn MR, Malanoski MP, Hetz SP, Rich NM. An external audit of laparoscopic cholecystectomy in the steady state performed in medical treatment facilities of the Department of Defense. Ann Surg 1996; 224:145–154.

45. Sadeghi-Nejad H, Kavoussi LR, Peters CA. Bowel injury in open technique laparoscopic cannula placement. Urology 1994; 43:559–560.

46. Kornfield EA, Sant GR, O'Leary MP. Minilaparotomy for laparoscopy: not a foolproof procedure. J Endourol 1994; 8:353–355.

47. Hanney RM, Carmalt HL, Merrett N, Tait N. Use of the Hasson cannula producing major vascular injury at laparoscopy. Surg Endosc 1999; 13:1238–1240.

48. Penfield AJ. How to prevent complications of open laparoscopy. J Reprod Med 1985; 30:660–663.

49. String A, Berber E, Foroutani A, Macho JR, Pearl JM, Siperstein AE. Use of the optical access trocar for safe and rapid entry in various laparoscopic procedures. Surg Endosc 2001; 15:570–573.

50. Marcovich R, Del Terzo MA, Wolf JS Jr. Comparison of transperitoneal laparoscopic access techniques: optiview visualizing trocar and Veress needle. J Endourol 2000; 14:175–179.

51. Vilos GA. Extracorporeal suturing of trocar-induced defects and vascular injuries in the abdominal wall during laparoscopy using a modified Veress needle. Obstet Gynecol 1995; 85:638–640.

52. Champault G, Cazacu F, Taffinder N. Serious trocar accidents in laparoscopic surgery: a French survey of 103,852 operations. Surg Laparosc Endosc 1996; 6:367–370.

53. Dixon M, Carrillo EH. Iliac vascular injuries during elective laparoscopic surgery. Surg Endosc 1999; 13:1230–1233.

54. Lantz PE, Smith JD. Fatal carbon dioxide embolism complicating attempted laparoscopic cholecystectomy—case report and literature review. J Forensic Sci 1994; 39:1468–1480.

55. Seidman DS, Nasserbakht F, Nezhat F, Nezhat, C, Nezhat C. Delayed recognition of iliac artery injury during laparoscopic surgery. Surg Endosc 1996; 10:1099–1101.

56. Golshani S, Simons AJ, Der R, Ortega AE. Necrotizing fasciitis following laparoscopic surgery. Surg Endosc 1996; 10:751–754.

57. Hurd WW, Pearl ML, DeLancey JO, Quint EH, Garnett B, Bude RO. Laparoscopic injury of abdominal wall blood vessels: a report of three cases. Obstet Gynecol 1993; 82:673–676.

58. Bakshi GK, Agrawal S, Shetty SV. A giant parietal wall hematoma: unusual complication of laparoscopic appendectomy. JSLS 2000; 4:255–257.

3

Major Vascular Injuries of Urologic Laparoscopic Surgery

PAUL YURKANIN

Southern Arizona Urologic Oncology
Tucson, Arizona, U.S.A.

EUGENE PARK

Urological Associates of Southern
Arizona, P.C, Tucson,
Arizona, U.S.A.

SANJAY RAMAKUMAR

University of Arizona Health Sciences
Center, Tucson, Arizona, U.S.A.

INTRODUCTION

Arterial vascular injuries associated with urologic laparoscopy are usually uncommon. However, they can be some of the most devastating problems encountered by the surgeon, resulting in unnecessary blood loss, poor visualization, conversion to an open surgical procedure, specific or multiple organ compromise/failure, shock, or ultimately death. These injuries may occur at any time during the operation, such as with trocar placement, tissue dissection, or isolation and ligation of vascular structures. They may be diagnosed intraoperatively or postoperatively. The key to these injuries is prevention with meticulous surgical skill and surgeon patience. However, when major arterial injuries occur, early recognition with a prompt and appropriate response is paramount to a successful outcome. The principles of managing significant venous injuries are similar to arterial injuries, with some minor differences outlined in this chapter.

REVIEW OF THE LITERATURE

Vascular injuries occur in approximately 1–3% of all urologic laparoscopic procedures and 0.5–3% are associated with uncontrollable hemorrhage (1–5). Hematoma formation requiring a transfusion and conversion to an open procedure secondary to bleeding are two of the most common complications (4,5). Injuries that have been reported or potentially may occur include laceration or transection of the aorta and vena cava (manuscript submitted) and any of its branches, inadvertent ligation of aortic branches, embolism or thrombosis of major aortic branches, and arteriovenous fistulas (1,2,4,6–8).

When immediately recognized, some major vascular complications may be treated laparoscopically depending upon the comfort level and experience of the surgeon (3,4,6). However, vascular injuries in general account for a large number of conversions from the laparoscopic to the open surgical approach (1–6). When a major arterial injury is not immediately recognized, certain postoperative findings may be indicative of the underlying problem. These include abdominal pain, nausea, vomiting, hypotension, absent pulses, detection of a new bruit, decreasing hematocrit, renal insufficiency, altered blood flow on Doppler ultrasonography, hematoma formation on computed tomography scanning, and either absent flow or extravasation of contrast on angiography (8,9).

However, it is apparent that the overall risk of all laparoscopic surgical complications decreases with increased surgical experience (2,5).

KEYS TO DIAGNOSIS

As previously mentioned, major arterial injuries may occur at any time during a laparoscopic procedure. Therefore, a high level of vigilance must be maintained throughout the entire operation in order to recognize these complications.

At the beginning of a laparoscopic procedure, access to the operative sight is obtained. This may involve Veress needle placement with eventual trocar placement. It is possible that either the Veress needle or a trocar may lacerate or transect the aorta or one of its branches. A Veress needle injury may be identified if the surgeon aspirates bright red blood or witnesses pulsatile blood flow through the needle. With either a Veress needle or trocar injury, hemorrhage or rapid abdominal distention may occur.

The majority of large arterial injuries occur during surgical dissection. These include the laceration, transection, and ligation of arteries. The injury may be immediately apparent with brisk bleeding noted or it may be delayed. Injuries that are not initially identified may be diagnosed later during the operation as time progresses. For example, a hematoma such as a mesenteric hematoma may be identified when a mesenteric vessel is injured. When there is inadvertent ligation of large arteries without adequate collateral circulation, organ compromise can occur. For example, with ligation of the superior mesenteric artery or splenic artery, bowel necrosis or a splenic infarct may occur.

Consideration must also be given to the specific nature of laparoscopic surgery. Special ligating clips, staple devices, and suture devices have been developed for laparoscopy. Like any mechanical device, these instruments may fail during key portions of the operation and lead to devastating consequences. Additionally, the pressure created from insufflation of the operative field may disguise bleeding vessels. Therefore, it is essential that near the completion of the procedure the insufflation pressure be decreased to less than 10 mmHg and inspection for persistent bleeding be performed.

Even with meticulous inspection at the completion of a procedure, an arterial injury may go unrecognized and not become manifest until the postoperative period. Therefore, as with all postoperative care, the surgeon must always be vigilant for these injuries. A patient may complain of generalized malaise, weakness, or nausea. Physical examination may demonstrate fever, tachycardia, hypotension, oliguria or anuria, ecchymosis, abdominal or pelvic distention or pain, a new bruit, or loss of previously palpable pulses. Laboratory studies may demonstrate an elevated white blood cell count, anemia, acidosis, electrolyte disturbances, elevated sedimentation rate, elevated lactate dehydrogenase, or renal insufficiency or failure. Radiographic tests may reveal hematoma formation, ongoing hemorrhage, loss of arterial blood flow, or an arteriovenous fistula.

If a major arterial injury is suspected in the postoperative period but is uncertain, diagnostic laparoscopy or open surgical exploration may be warranted for confirmation.

MANAGEMENT STRATEGIES

When a Veress needle punctures a large artery and significant bleeding is identified, the stopcock should be closed and the needle left in place. It should not be twisted or further manipulated as this may turn a puncture into a laceration. With the needle in place, an immediate laparotomy is necessary in order to identify and repair the injury.

A trocar injury to a large artery is treated in a similar fashion as a Veress needle injury. The injury may be recognized initially with brisk bleeding or may not be identified until later if bleeding is confined to the retroperitoneum. Once the injury is recognized, a laparotomy is performed in order to repair the injury (6).

As previously mentioned, most arterial injuries will occur during surgical dissection. The key to these injuries is early recognition. Once the injury is recognized, a decision is made whether to repair the injury or ligate the vessel. In order to make the appropriate decision, one must consider anatomy, collateral circulation, and overall vascular status of the patient. Aortic, common iliac, or external iliac arterial injuries need to be repaired. Internal iliac artery injuries should be repaired if they are proximal to the superior gluteal artery. When the injury is distal to the superior gluteal artery, consideration can be given to ligation of the internal iliac artery if good collateral flow exists from the contralateral artery (10).

Visceral arterial injuries can be devastating and are associated with a high level of mortality. Injury to the celiac axis, superior mesenteric artery, or inferior mesenteric artery can present with bleeding or a mesenteric hematoma. It is recommended that superior mesenteric artery injuries be primarily repaired. Consideration can be given to ligation of the celiac axis or inferior mesenteric artery if adequate collateral circulation exists. Otherwise, repair of these injuries must be performed (11).

Renal artery injuries are approached individually. If a kidney is to be removed, then a renal artery injury may result in earlier vessel ligation than anticipated. However, if kidney preservation is desired (i.e., solitary kidney or partial nephrectomy) then the artery must be repaired.

Splenic artery injuries are also approached individually with usually ligation or splenectomy. Rarely are these injuries repaired.

Before repairing a major arterial injury, the basic principles of vascular surgery must be understood. Once an injury occurs and is identified, hemostasis is obtained by thorough proximal and distal control of the vessel. Both the anterior and posterior aspects of the vessel are inspected to survey for injury extent. A decision is then made with regard to ligation or repair as outlined above. A low threshold for obtaining intraoperative vascular surgery consultation is paramount as patient safety is the first priority.

When repairing lacerations or transactions, the normal caliber of the artery must be maintained. A narrowed vessel has reduced flow and is at increased risk for thrombosis. Lacerations can be closed using monofilament polypropylene suture in either a continuous (i.e., large vessel) or interrupted (i.e., medium or small vessels) fashion. Vein or Gore-Tex patch grafts are used as needed. Sutures should always be passed in the direction of blood flow when possible to limit the likelihood of intimal elevation.

For a complete transection, an end-to-end anastomosis is most desirable, with an end-to-side anastomosis the next best alternative. The advenitia of the vessel is removed from the site where the repair is to take place. Care is taken not to injure the intima. Double-armed corner sutures are placed 180° apart and tied. Sutures are then placed, beginning at the corners and working toward the middle. The vessel can be flushed with a dilute heparin solution at the beginning and just before placing the final suture in order to decrease the likelihood of air emboli. Systemic heparinization is considered if there is total arterial flow occlusion to the lower extremity for a prolonged period of time during injury repair (7).

With laparoscopy, the surgeon has additional tools within his or her armamentarium to combat vascular injuries. In some instances, electrocautery or clips may be all that is needed to obtain hemostasis. However, care must be taken not to narrow or occlude vital vessels. A Foley catheter loaded with a catheter guide may be passed through a trocar, positioned into a laceration, and then the balloon inflated in order to tamponade bleeding. Furthermore, the extremely experienced minimally invasive surgeon may be able to laparoscopically repair large artery lacerations with skillful suturing (6).

When a major arterial injury is not diagnosed until the postoperative period, the management approach may be different. Certain injuries can be observed with serial hematocrit assessments and transfusions as necessary. A decision for radiologic or surgical intervention can be made based upon the patient's clinical course. When there is arterial occlusion secondary to thrombus formation or embolization, the need for anticoagulation, thromboembolic therapy, or revascularization is determined based upon the individual case.

In addition to the strategies described above, major venous injuries can be managed by simple tamponade before identification and repair or ligation. Through a 12 mm port, a small laparotomy pad can be introduced and then applied to the bleeding site. The insufflation pressure can be raised and the area is compressed for a few minutes. Slow withdrawal of the pad with suction instruments nearby will usually reveal the source of bleeding. Alternatively, during hand-assisted laparoscopy, a large laparotomy pad is kept within the abdomen throughout the case or is placed through the handport when needed.

A unique complication that may not arise until later in the postoperative period is an arteriovenous fistula, which can result from en mass staple ligation of major arteries and veins together. This complication can be relatively asymptomatic or may cause significant cardiovascular compromise. Depending upon the size of the fistula and its impact on overall patient health, the fistula may be observed or treated. Treatment options include angiographic embolization or surgical exploration with repair or ligation.

PREVENTION TECHNIQUES

Major arterial injuries can be some of the most devastating injuries encountered in laparoscopic surgery. The key to these injuries is to prevent them from occurring. This is best done with a firm knowledge and understanding of vascular anatomy, precision and delicacy with Veress needle and trocar placement, meticulous surgical dissection, and conversion to an open procedure when necessary before encountering an injury. Patient safety is of utmost importance and should always be the first consideration in the surgeon's mind during any procedure.

KEY POINTS

- Major arterial injuries are rare, but significantly impact procedure success and patient outcome.
- Prevention is paramount.
- Intraoperative diagnosis by identifying hemorrhage or a hematoma; look for hemorrhage under low pressure conditions at the end of the procedure.

- Tamponade may help identify the location of vascular injury.
- Postoperative diagnosis through patient complaint, physical exam, laboratory tests, or diagnostic study.
- Determine if reasonable to ligate the vessel or if repair is necessary.
- Laparoscopic repair may be feasible, but open conversion is likely.
- Vascular surgeon or interventional radiology consultation when necessary.
- Patient safety is the main priority.

REFERENCES

1. Gill IS, Kavoussi LR, Clayman RV, Ehrlich R, Evans R, Fuchs G, Gershman A, Hulbert JC, McDougall EM, Rosenthal T, Schuessler WW, Shepard T. Complications of laparoscopic nephrectomy in 185 patients: a multi-institutional review. J Urol 1995; 154:479–483.

2. Peters CA. Complications in pediatric urological laparoscopy: results of a survey. J Urol 1996; 155:1070–1073.

3. Thomas R, Steele R, Ahuja S. Complications of urological laparoscopy: a standardized 1 institution experience. J Urol 1996; 156:469–471.

4. Soulie M, Seguin P, Richeux L, Mouly P, Vazzoler N, Pontonnier F, Plante P. Urological complications of laparoscopic surgery: experience with 350 procedures at a single center. J Urol 2001; 165:1960–1963.

5. Cadeddu JA, Wolfe JS, Nakada S, Chen R, Shalhav A, Bishoff JT, Hamilton B, Schulam PG, Dunn M, Hoenig D, Fabrizio M, Hedican S, Averch TD. Complications of laparoscopic procedures after concentrated training in urological laparoscopy. J Urol 2001; 166:2109–2111.

6. Kavoussi LR. Complications of laparoscopic surgery. In: Bishoff JT, Kavoussi LR, eds. Atlas of Laparoscopic Retroperitoneal Surgery. Philadelphia: Saunders, 2000:237–253.

7. Macfarlane MT, Smith RB. Management of vascular complications. In: Taneja SS, Smith RB, Ehrlich RM, eds. Compli-

cations of Urologic Surgery Prevention and Management. Philadelphia: Saunders, 2001:167–176.

8. Yaycioglu O, Ramakumar S, Kavoussi LR, Jarrett TW. Early repeated exploration after laparoscopic urologic surgery: comparison of clinical, radiologic, and surgical findings. Urology 2002; 59:190–194.

9. Britt LD, Weireter LJ, Cole FJ. Newer diagnostic modalities for vascular injuries. Surg Clin North Am 2001; 81:1263–1277.

10. Lee JT, Bongard FS. Iliac vessel injuries. Surg Clin North Am 2002; 82:21–43.

11. Asensio JA, Forno W, Roldan G, Petrone P, Rojo E, Ceballos J, Wang C, Costaglioli B, Romero J, Tillou A, Carmody I, Shoemaker WC, Berne TV. Visceral Vascular Injuries. Surg Clin North Am 2002; 82:1–17.

4

Stapler Malfunction and Management

DAVID Y. CHAN

The James Buchanan Brady Urological Institute,
Johns Hopkins Medical Institutions,
Baltimore, Maryland, U.S.A.

INTRODUCTION

Laparoscopic nephrectomy has evolved since the first reported case by Clayman et al. (1) and is an acceptable alternative for live renal donation (2,3) and the treatment of benign (4,5) and malignant disease (6,7). Early challenges the procedure involved the controlled ligation and division of the renal artery and renal vein. The GIA was developed and allowed for safe controlled ligation and division of the intended vessel. Failure of the device, however, can be associated with severe consequences including emergent conversion to an open procedure and the possible loss of renal allograft in cases of live kidney donation. The majority of problems, however, can be avoided with careful application and recognition. Many failures, especially if recognized prior to release of the device, can be managed without conversion to an open procedure.

SCOPE OF THE PROBLEM

Two recent reviews have examined prevalence of stapler malfunctions (8,9). Primary device failure is an uncommon event. Both Deng et al. and Chan et al. reported a primary device failure of 0.3% and 0.2%, respectively. In most cases, the device failures are preventable and usually associated with surgeon or surgical team error (Table 1).

Deng et al. also searched the U. S. Food and Drug Administration Manufacturer and User Facility Device Experience Database (MAUDE) and found 60 reported laparoscopic endovascular stapler problems in 55 patients. The prevalence was not calculated as the database is voluntary and does not report or estimate the number of staplers and reloads used. The malfunctions noted include (1) defect in the unused product, (2) abnormal jaw closure, (3) problem with deployment, (4) problem with stapler removal, (5) staple line bleeding, and (6) incomplete transection of tissue.

Table 1 Etiology of Failures

Etiology	Number
Preventable causes	7
Device deployed over previous surgical clip	5
Caval injury from entrapment in sliding mechanism of device	1
Incomplete transection of vessel	1
Primary instrument failure	3
Missing row of staples	1
Failure of ligation	2

PREVENTION

The most important first step in management of stapler malfunction is prevention and early recognition. Prior to application, the stapler device should be carefully inspected to ensure proper loading, alignment, and the presence of staples. This will prevent problems with the product and avoid misalignment and firing. In one case reported, there was absence of proximal row of staples. This resulted in immediate laparotomy.

Similarly, the surgeon should use surgical clips judiciously and keep an accurate count of surgical clips near the hilum. This will prevent and reduce the risk of entrapping clips within the jaws of stapler. Staple clip entrapment can lead to misalignment and incomplete stapling and premature transection. The Ligasure device (Valley Labs, Boulder, CO) has been used for control of small vessels around the hilum. This device has been approved for ligation of vessels less than 7 mm and obviates the use of metallic elements that could interfere with the stapler device closure and application.

Proper GIA placement is also important to prevent incomplete vessel transection or injury to adjacent tissue from the sliding mechanism of the proximal portion of the GIA device. If the jaws of the stapler do not close completely, the device should not be deployed. The stapler should be release and reexamined. If the stapler will not fire easy, do not force the stapler. This may be a sign of an empty stapler cartilage. One should not use excessive force to override the lockout mechanism. This will result in tissue transection without ligation.

If the activation of the device is not smooth, GIA misfire should be suspected. If malfunction is recognized early, prior to release of the stapler device, placement of surgical clip or secondary GIA device proximally may be possible for vascular control. It is often prudent to pause after firing the stapler device and inspect for bleeding prior to release of the stapler.

If bleeding is noted, the GIA device should be kept in place until definitive management has been established. Surgeon experience ultimately mandates the final decision to either convert to an open procedure or to try to control the

Table 2 Management

Management	Number
Laparoscopic	8
Proximal placement of GIA	3
Intracorporeal repair of vessel, proximal clip or suturing	5
Laparotomy	2

problem laparoscopically. There should be, however, a low threshold for laparotomy with living donor nephrectomy where both donor and renal allograft are at risk.

The early recognition of malfunction prior to release of the device is quintessential in the ability to manage these complications laparoscopically. If bleeding does ensue, the surgeon may try to control bleeding with direct pressure and improved exposure. An additional 10–12 mm trocar may be placed to help with laparoscopic management. Most failures can be managed without conversion to an open procedure by prompt recognition, and immediate control of bleeding with direct pressure. Subsequent vessel ligation can often be achieved by either intracorporeal suturing techniques or with the aid of such devices as EndoStitch (US Surgical, Norwalk, CT) and fabricated "knots" (LapraTy, Ethicon Endosurgery, Cincinnati, OH), or placement of vascular clips. An additional application of another GIA or TA stapler proximal to the malfunction is often feasible. Prompt recognition allows for correction of the situation without significant bleeding.

If bleeding is excessive or laparoscopic management is not possible, there should be early consideration of open laparotomy for definitive repair. Again, surgeon experience and comfort level will dictate the most efficient and effective management options (Table 2).

CONCLUSIONS

Use of the GIA is standard for control of renal hilar vessels during laparoscopic nephrectomy. Failure of the device is uncommon and is usually related to preventable causes. Most malfunctions can be handled without conversion to an open procedure and the incidence of primary device failure is very low (<0.3%). The use of the GIA device for vascular control is safe and effective.

KEY POINTS

- Judicious use and accurate count of surgical clips near the hilum;
- ensure absence of clips within the jaws of the GIA;
- proper GIA placement to prevent incomplete vessel transection or injury to adjacent tissue from sliding mechanism of the proximal portion of the GIA device;
- suspect GIA misfire if activation of device is not smooth;
- if malfunction is recognized early, i.e., prior to release of device, placement of surgical clips or secondary GIA device proximally may be possible for vascular control;
- if bleeding ensues during nephrectomy for benign and malignant disease, try to control bleeding with direct pressure and improved exposure;
- low threshold for laparotomy with live donor nephrectomy where both donor and renal allograft are at risk;
- surgeon experience mandates the final decision to either convert to an open procedure or to try to control the problem laparoscopically.

REFERENCES

1. Clayman RV, Kavoussi LR, Soper NJ, Dierks SM, Meretyk S, Darcy MD, Roemer FD, Pingleton ED, Thomson PG, Long SR. Laparoscopic nephrectomy: initial case report. J Urol 1991; 146(2):278–282.

2. Fabrizio MD, Ratner LE, Kavoussi LR. Laparoscopic live donor nephrectomy: pro. Urology 1999; 53(4):665–667.

3. Flowers JL, Jacobs S, Cho E, Morton A, Rosenberger WF, Evans D, Imbembo AL, Bartlett ST. Comparison of open and

laparoscopic live donor nephrectomy. Ann Surg 1997; 226(4):483–489; discussion 489–490.

4. Hoenig DM, McDougall EM, Shalhav AL, Elbahnasy AM, Clayman RV. Laparoscopic ablation of peripelvic renal cysts. J Urol 1997; 158(4):1345–1348.

5. Chen RN, Moore RG, Kavoussi LR. Laparoscopic pyeloplasty. Indications, technique, and long-term outcome. Urol Clin North Am 1998; 25(2):323–330.

6. Cadeddu JA, Ono Y, Clayman RV, Barrett PH, Janetschek G, Fentie DD, McDougall EM, Moore RG, Kinukawa T, Elbahnasy AM, Nelson JB, Kavoussi LR. Laparoscopic nephrectomy for renal cell cancer: evaluation of efficacy and safety: a multicenter experience. Urology 1998; 52(5):773–777.

7. Jarrett TW, Cadeddu JA, Fabrizio MD, Chan DY, Nelson JB, Kavoussi LR. Laparoscopy in the treatment of upper tract transitional cell carcinoma. J Endourol 1999; 13(S1):A66.

8. Deng DY, Meng MV, Nguyen HT, Bellman GC, Stoller ML. Laparoscopic linear cutting stapler failure. Urology 2002; 60(3):415–419; discussion 419–420.

9. Chan D, Bishoff JT, Ratner L, Kavoussi LR, Jarrett TW. Endovascular gastrointestinal stapler device malfunction during laparoscopic nephrectomy: early recognition and management. J Urol 2000; 164(2):319–321.

5

Bowel Injury

TIMOTHY M. PHILIPS and JAY T. BISHOFF
Endourology Section, Department of Urology,
Wilford Hall Medical Center, Lackland Air Force
Base, Texas, U.S.A.

INTRODUCTION

Laparoscopy was initially performed by Kelling in 1901 (1), and now almost a century later this technique has gained global popularity and widespread use for many procedures in multiple specialties. Because laparoscopic surgery offers benefits over open surgery including less postoperative pain, shorter convalescence, and improved cosmesis, it has replaced laparotomy in many instances as the preferred route of treating surgical pathology. Surveys of complications from laparoscopy have been published for abdominal and pelvic procedures. Intestinal injury represents a rare but potentially fatal complication of any abdominal procedure. In laparoscopic patients, the signs and symptoms of bowel injury may be

49

different from that seen after traditional laparotomy. The following presents a review of the literature with respect to laparoscopic bowel injury. Keys to the diagnosis of bowel injury will be emphasized as well as the subsequent management strategies. Prevention techniques and key points will be highlighted at the end.

REVIEW OF THE LITERATURE

In a recent review, the combined incidence of reported laparoscopic bowel injury was 0.13% (266/205,969) (2). Small bowel injuries accounted for 58% of intestinal injuries, followed by colon 32% and stomach 7%. When considering only injuries related to establishing primary entry access, injuries to the small bowel reportedly account for 25% of all laparoscopic complications with the colon and stomach accounting for 12% and 1.6% of entry access injuries, respectively (3). In smaller series, the incidence of bowel abrasion without perforation is reported to occur in 0.6% of patients (2).

The majority of reported injuries (69%) were not recognized at the time of surgery (2). In fact, punctures to the small and large bowel are significantly more likely than other injuries to go unrecognized for 24 hr to several days and account for 76% of injuries with a 24-hr or greater delay in diagnosis (3). The reported time to presentation of unrecognized bowel injury after surgery depends upon the segment involved and the etiology of the injury. Small bowel injuries are recognized on an average of 4.5 days after surgery (range 2–14 days) and large bowel injuries recognized on an average of 5.4 days following surgery (range 1–29 days) (2). This is especially important given the reported 20% mortality of laparoscopic small bowel injury (3). When considering all complications with a delay in diagnosis of greater than 24-hr of which bowel injuries account for 76%, the mortality increases to 26%. Duodenal injury, in particular, carries an exceedingly high mortality, reported as high as 75% in some studies (4).

Fifty percent of bowel injuries are reportedly caused by electrocautery and 32% occurred during Veress needle or trocar insertion (2). Thermal bowel injuries typically present later than nonthermal injuries due to delayed breakdown of the intestinal wall at the injury site. Blunt and sharp dissections, as well as injuries from grasping forceps, are certainly known causes of bowel injury. Isolated cases of intestinal injury attributable to ultrasonic shears and suction irrigators have also been reported (5,6). In one study, 34% of all laparoscopic complications occurred during the set-up phase (creation of pneumoperitoneum and installation of trocars), emphasizing the importance of this portion of a laparoscopic procedure (6).

Commonly reported technical errors during trocar insertion include inadequate stabilization of the abdominal wall, inadequate size of trocar site incision, excessive resistance to trocar insertion, misdirected or poorly controlled force directed by the surgeon along the axis of the trocar (8). El-Banna et al. (4) found that 50% of the bowel injuries occurred at the hands of experienced surgeons who had performed >100 laparoscopic cases. This was attributed to the experienced surgeon's likelihood of performing more advanced cases, especially in patients with previous abdominal surgeries, as well as a higher threshold for converting to laparotomy.

KEYS TO DIAGNOSIS

In laparoscopic surgery, if a bowel injury is not identified intraoperatively, it can be subsequently difficult to identify this iatrogenic injury in the postoperative period. Since the majority of injuries are not recognized during surgery, they present at variable times during the postoperative period. The diagnosis of a complication in the postsurgical abdomen is often challenging. Subtle and possibly serious changes can be masked by postoperative pain, narcotic medications, and antibiotics, creating a diagnostic dilemma for even the most experienced surgeon. Typically, postoperative peritonitis from an anastomotic leak or perforated viscus would be expected to present with ileus, worsening abdominal pain, abdominal rigidity, leukocytosis with a left shift, fever, large volume fluid requirements, followed by tachycardia and hypotension (9,10). However, the signs and symptoms of bowel injury in postoperative laparoscopy patients often present in a different fashion compared to those typically associated with intra-abdominal processes and sepsis. Patients should always be informed of the small risk of visceral injury in laparoscopic surgery and should be instructed on how they recognize these early symptoms of injury so that definitive diagnosis and prompt intervention can be employed.

The most opportune time to diagnose a bowel injury is at the time of occurrence. Overt signs of bowel injury include the detection of foul smelling gas or greenish fluid at the time of surgery or from the open end of a Veress needle or trocar upon the initial establishment of pneumoperitoneum (11). If this occurs, but there is still some doubt of a bowel injury, syringe aspiration can be used. If an injury is still not detected, insertion of the laparoscope at this time may allow the visualization of bowel mucosa. Insufflation pressures that become elevated very quickly after establishing pneumoperitoneum are also concerning for a possible cannulation of the small bowel with a trocar or Veress needle (12). If there is slight leakage without obvious extravasation, the laceration is unfortunately likely to remain unrecognized intraoperatively. Moving small bowel loops and the greater momentum tend to hide the defect and even close the leakage temporarily (13). Despite the initial clues, bowel injury can still go unnoticed during the initial operation.

In a review of the literature by Bishoff et al., of 10 patients with bowel perforation four were unrecognized at the time of surgery (Table 1). The initial presenting complaint in all patients with unrecognized injury was persistent and relatively increased trocar site pain at a single trocar site, without significant erythema or purulent drainage (2). At the time of subsequent exploration, the painful trocar site was found to be closest to the injured bowel segment. In this group, symptoms were initially nonspecific including abdominal distension and diarrhea. However, ileus, diffuse abdominal pain, nausea, and vomiting were uncommon findings (Table 2). Surprisingly, only one patient displayed a fever

Table 1 Summary of 10 Patients with Laparoscopic Bowel Injury

Patient	Procedure	Injury site	Injury type	Repair	Complication	Time to recognition
Injuries recognized at the time of the procedure						
1	Nephrectomy	Small bowel	Dissection abrasion	None	Abscess and fistula	2 Weeks
2	Pyeloplasty	Colon	Dissection abrasion	Oversewn	None	
3	PLND	Colon	Dissection abrasion	Oversewn	None	
4	PLND	Colon	Dissection abrasion	Oversewn	None	
5	Pyeloplasty	Colon	Dissection abrasion	Oversewn	None	
6	PLND	Colon	Burn	Oversewn	None	
Injuries unrecognized at the time of surgery presenting in the early postoperative period						
7	Nephrectomy	Colon	Closure perforation	Drain	Enterocutaneousfistula	POD 10
8	PLND	Colon	Scissor perforation	None	Sepsis, Death	POD 4
9	Cholecystectomy	Duodenal	Scissor perforation	Laparotomy	Necrotizing fasciitis	POD 3
10	PLND	Colon	Thermal perforation	Laparotomy	Sepsis, death	POD 3

PLND = pelvic lymph node dissection; POD = postoperative day.

Table 2 Unrecognized Laparoscopic Bowel Injury Patients Presenting Signs and Symptoms

		Patient number			
Signs and symptoms	#1	#7	#8	#9	#10
Trocar pain	Y	Y	Y	Y	Y
Abdominal distension	Y	Y	Y	Y	Y
Leukopenia	Y	N	Y	Y	Y
Diarrhea	Y	N	Y	Y	Y
Cardiovascular collapse	N	N	Y	Y	Y
Ileus	N	N	N	N	Y
Abdominal pain	N	N	N	N	N
Leukocytosis	N	N	N	N	N
Fever > 101	N	N	N	Y	N
Nausea	Y	N	N	Y	Y
Vomiting	N	N	N	Y	Y

N = patient *did not* present with this sign or symptom; Y = patient *did* present with this sign or symptom.

greater than 38°C, and none of the patients developed a leukocytosis or peritoneal signs. In fact, all but one patient displayed leukopenia. Two patients with colon injuries after staging pelvic lymph node dissection had rapid onset of sepsis and died within 4 days of surgery. Both patients had a clinical presentation that was atypical for an intraabdominal abscess including fever <38°C, no peritoneal signs, persistent bowel sounds, diarrhea and leukopenia in the postoperative period.

These findings are particularly interesting, in that the majority of patients did not present in the typical fashion. Instead, these patients had low-grade temperatures and all but one patient displayed leukopenia (1000–4000/u L). Furthermore, ileus, abdominal pain, nausea, and vomiting were uncommon complaints. While patients reported generalized discomfort consistent with surgery, the initial presenting complaint in all patients with unrecognized bowel injury was persistent and relatively extreme trocar site pain at the site closest to the bowel injury. No purulence or erythema was noted at any of the trocar sites. The exact nature of the trocar site pain is unknown, but likely represents local irritation from bowel contents. In each case, symptoms included abdominal distension and diarrhea in the face of persistent bowel sounds and absence of severe abdominal pain or peritoneal signs.

Others have described a similar presentation of bowel injury in the laparoscopic patient. Thompson and Wheeless reported on five patients with unrecognized bowel injuries after laparoscopic sterilization. These patients presented within 3 days after the procedure with nausea, diarrhea, anorexia, low-grade fever, persistent bowel sounds, and a low or normal white blood cell count (4000–10,000). In this series, only two of the patients presented with ileus and peritoneal signs. All of the patients underwent laparotomy for drainage of an abscess and with resection and repair of the damaged bowel segment (14).

Small bowel perforation presenting in the postoperative period with only persistent excessive external fluid leak from the periumbilical area after laparoscopic surgery, with no drainage from other incisional sites, has also been reported (15).

The exact etiology for the unusual presentation of laparoscopic bowel injury compared to open surgery is not currently known. Iatrogenic internal to external canalization between the small intestine and the skin has been proposed as a possible mechanism for the masked clinical signs and symptoms of small intestinal injury in laparoscopic surgery (15). Other series suggest that the postoperative response to bowel injury in laparoscopic surgery may be different from that of the open patient (2). The lower immune and metabolic stimulus that is caused by laparoscopic surgery may allow a more rapid progression toward sepsis before the natural homeostatic responses have occurred. The possibility that laparoscopic surgery produces less of a metabolic or immune response compared to open surgery has been explored. The severity of surgical injury is a major determinant of the degree of the immunologicaland metabolic reactions, which follow in the postoperative period (16).

Laparoscopic surgery is accomplished in the absence of a large skin incision, which in many cases is the site of maximum trauma. Less tissue destruction may result in less stimulation of acute-phase reactions and consequently may reduce the postsurgical metabolic and cytokine response. This difference may account for the unusual signs and symptoms seen in patients with laparoscopic bowel injury. Interleukin-6 (IL-6) is known to be a marker of tissue damage and is involved in the modulation of local inflammation and systemic acute-phase response resulting in synthesis of acute-phase proteins such as C-reactive protein (17,18). Whether or not laparoscopic surgery changes this response when compared to open surgery is controversial. There have been multiple reports comparing postoperative IL-6 levels after laparoscopic vs. open cholecystectomy. Most of the studies indicate that laparoscopic surgery was associated with significantly lower postoperative IL-6 responses compared with open surgery (19–21). Mealy et al. (22) found reduced levels of C-reactive proteins in laparoscopy vs. open cholecystectomy. In contrast, McMahon et al. (23) found no reduction in interleukin-6 or C-reactive proteins in a similar trial comparing open and laparoscopic cholecystectomy patients. Harmon et al. (24) compared serum IL-6 levels in patients who underwent laparoscopic colectomy to open colectomy levels and found that IL-6 levels were significantly lower in the laparoscopy group during the first 24 hr after surgery (24).

Failure to recognize and promptly treat a bowel injury results in a high rate of morbidity and mortality. Computerized tomography is indicated in laparoscopic patients with clinical findings suspicious for bowel injury in the early postoperative period and can reliably identify bowel perforation, postoperative bleeding, urinoma, and urinary obstruction (25). Plain upright or decubitus abdominal films have also proven reliable for the diagnosis of free intraabdominal air as a marker for bowel injury in the postoperative laparoscopic patient, such that the presence of free air 48–72 hr after laparoscopy may indicate the presence of a bowel injury (4). The laparoscopic surgeon must use clinical judgment, but if a patient is not progressing as would be expected at the 48 hr mark, then it is prudent to obtain a CT with oral and intravenous contrast to rule out bowel injury. The morbidity will increase dramatically after this point if diagnosis is delayed.

MANAGEMENT STRATEGIES

When a bowel perforation is recognized, immediate repair is indicated during that initial laparoscopic procedure. Several reports have shown the safety of laparoscopic repair and avoidance of colostomy even in the presence of rectal injury (26). Nezhat et al. reported on enterotomies repaired laparoscopically in 26 patients (small bowel—nine, colon—four, rectal—13) who preoperatively had mechanical and antibiotic bowel preparation. They reported no complications following laparoscopic enterotomy repair and all patients were discharged within 3 days (27). Injuries that present in the postoperative period will require open laparotomy in almost every case. In the review of the literature, 80% of late laparoscopic bowel injuries presenting in the postoperative period were managed with laparotomy (2). Other patients with diagnosed bowel injures were managed with total parenteral nutrition and percutaneous drainage or expectantly in the face of sepsis and cardiovascular collapse. In that review, 3% of patients (8/266) were reported to have died as a direct result of their unrecognized bowel injury. In a review by El-Banna et al. (4), immediately identified injuries to the small bowel and large bowel segments were repaired with good results. However, injuries with a delay in diagnosis usually required exteriorization of the injured segment and subsequent repair while one patient with an injury to the ascending colon required colostomy and drainage with interval colostomy takedown.

PREVENTION TECHNIQUES

Given that a significant percentage of bowel injuries occur while establishing primary entry access, this a crucial time during any laparoscopic procedure to institute safe strategies for injury prevention. Even after the exclusion of well-known causal factors such as inadequate instrumentation, poor technique, or insufficient training, there is still a substantial risk of bowel perforation mainly attributable to abdominal adhesions.

Many advocate that the best way to avoid visceral injury during trocar insertion is to use the open Hasson technique, whereby the trocar is inserted into the peritoneal cavity under direct-vision prior to the establishment of pneumoperitoneum. This has been especially advocated in very thin or obese individuals, in pediatric patients, and in patients who have had previous abdominal surgery (3). However, despite placement of trocars under direct vision with the Hasson technique, a continued bowel injury incidence of 0.06% has been reported (8) and multiple studies have documented no statistical difference in bowel injury rates when compared to closed techniques.

If a closed technique is used, the first trocar should be placed at a site remote from previous abdominal incisions with a high likelihood of underlying adhesions (8). In these cases, a previously established pneumoperitoneum through the use of a Veress needle or mechanical splinting should be used, and the axial force on the trocar should be controlled to avoid contact of the trocar tip with viscera or the retroperitoneum (8). The trocar incision site should be large enough to allow the trocar to enter without the edge being trapped by the skin, which can suddenly give way during insertion and injure underlying structures.

Alternative sites for the insertion of the Veress needle have been proposed to include a point located 3 cm inferior to the costal arch in the left mid-clavicular line (Palmer's point) (28). This site is usually free of adhesions, even in previously operated patients. To compliment this technique, more recently microlaparoscopes have been introduced that can be advanced through the outer sheath of a matching Veress needle. These laparoscopes have optics sufficient for diagnostic purposes and can be used to inspect the peritoneal cavity to include the underside of the anterior abdominal wall. As a viable means for the assessment of adhesions, the microlaparoscope can be used to directly visualize the insertion of the primary trocar through an appropriate site in the anterior abdominal wall (29). However, it must be noted that to date there has not been a documented decrease in the incidence of bowel injury using this technique.

One novel design intended to avoid visceral injury is the direct-view trocar. The laparoscope and cannula are inserted as a unit, and the surgeon can see the tissues as the trocar passes through them. Presumably, the surgeon would be able to see a viscus early enough to stop short of perforating it. Although there are claims that this device is safer than conventional cutting trocars, they have not become popular (8).

A through and through perforation of small bowel adherent to the anterior abdominal wall can occur without the surgeon's knowledge. If a trocar is placed completely through a viscus, the operator will not see the damage, as it will be behind the camera. If a Veress needle is put through a loop of bowel and enters the peritoneal cavity, it will test as being properly placed. The surgeon should be able to see this complication by placing the camera through another port and inspecting the Veress needle insertion site. As a result, this maneuver has been recommended at the beginning of every procedure.

Any patient undergoing laparoscopy should have an orogastric tube inserted to decrease gastric distention and avoid gastric injury during Veress needle and trocar placement. A bowel preparation in some patients may also be useful in decreasing soilage of the peritoneal cavity in the event of bowel injury, by facilitating operative maneuvers, and by increasing the size of the intraperitoneal free space (11). Trocar placement should be avoided near scars from previous abdominal surgery.

An additional source of intestinal injury during laparoscopy and thus an area for secondary prevention is intraoperative intestinal abrasions. While most series report only bowel perforations, the recent series by Bishoff et al. (2) included serosal abrasions as bowel injuries because one patient who had a seemingly insignificant and thus unrepaired serosal abrasion during intestinal mobilization later developed an abscess and enterocutaneous fistula. This abscess was determined to be in the area of the known abrasion. Subsequent to this event, all serosal abrasions regardless of severity were repaired by over sewing the area to protect from fistulization and abscess formation.

Over half of laparoscopic bowel injuries reported in the literature is reported to be caused by electrocautery insult. Thermal injury can be prevented with vigilant surveillance of cautery contact points during dissection. Energy should be applied to the tip only when in contact with target tissues. Furthermore, the laparoscopic surgeon should avoid application of monopolar electricity to ductlike strands of tissue that may be attached to bowel. Waye et al. demonstrated the ease of raising the temperature of tissue many centimeters from the operative site by using monopolar electrocautery. They were able to show that if a temperature differential of 30°C was reached for only 2 sec, tissue death occurred (2). Additionally, cautery effect has been demonstrated after an electrical burn in bowel as far as 5 cm away from the site of injury (30).

Since only 10–15% of the entire laparoscopic instrument is visualized during surgery, breaks in the integrity of the insulated coating and capacitive coupling can occur along the shaft of the instrument or through a metal trocar resulting in thermal injury to bowel out of the surgeons view. Capacitive coupling has been shown to occur along the shaft of some instruments where the insulation coat is relatively thin. This stray energy may be responsible for otherwise unrecognized, unintentional injury during monopolar laparoscopic electrosurgery (31,32). The laparoscopic surgeon should be aware of the warning signs of metal to metal arching during surgery, such as involuntary contraction of abdominal muscles, hissing sounds within the trocar or "lightening" artifacts on monitors and electrical equipment (33). Also a reduction in the expected electrosurgical effect at a given power setting and energy mode may indicate that some of the electroenergy had dissipated away from the tip of the electrode. An increase in the power output should be avoided and a check of system integrity should be made. The occurrence of cautery injury outside the surgeon's field of view can be minimized through the use of active electrode monitoring (AEM) devices or insulation scanners for monopolar instruments and bipolar electrocautery. The Electroscope^{TM} AEM system (Electroscope, Inc., Boulder, CO) includes a unique set of laparoscopic instruments that are simultaneously connected to a standard electrocautery machine and to a separate device that continuously searches for stray energy escaping along the shaft of the instrument and deactivates the electrosurgical generator before injury can occur. The integrity of the insulated coating on the shaft of laparoscopic instruments can also be determined on the back table, prior to placing the instrument into the patient, using the InsulScan (Medline Industries, Inc., Mundelein, IL).

As a result of the known complications of electrocautery in laparoscopic surgery, the use of the ultrasonic coagulating shears has been advocated as producing less thermal injury in animal models than electrocautery during laparoscopic dissection (11). Ultrasonic dissection separates tissues with a cavitational effect and achieves hemostasis by disrupting protein structure and forming a coagulum, producing minimal local heat. Though this intuitively results in a safer means of tissue dissection as opposed to electrocautery, the exact incidence of bowel or other visceral injury attributable to the use of ultrasonic dissection techniques in not known. While electricity is not produced at the tip of the harmonic shears, the tips of the shears do become hot during coagulation and can injure bowel segments if used for dissection following activation. There are reported cases of bowel injury using ultrasonic techniques (5,34).

Laparoscopic bowel injury is a rare complication with potentially devastating consequences if not promptly recognized and treated. In the laparoscopic patient, the presenting signs and symptoms may differ from classical teachings about the acute abdomen. Immediate repair of injuries in the operating room is recommended. The diagnosis of an unrecognized bowel injury may be difficult in the postoperative period. Prompt imaging with a CT scan of the abdomen and pelvis is a valuable diagnostic tool and immediate surgical exploration is required when a bowel injury has been identified.

KEY POINTS

- Bowel injury occurs in less than 1% of laparoscopic cases.
- Small bowel is the most commonly injured bowel segment and electrocautery is the most common cause of injury.

- The clinical presentation following bowel injury can be confusing.
- Patients with unrecognized bowel injury typically have severe pain at one trocar site, abdominal distension, diarrhea, and leukopenia. They rarely present with ileus, peritoneal signs, and leukocytosis.
- Failure to recognize the presence of bowel injury in the postoperative laparoscopic patient can rapidly lead to septic shock and death.
- Minor appearing serosal abrasions can develop into full thickness bowel injuries and should be over sewn when recognized.
- When bowel injury is suspected, CT scan can assist with the diagnosis. Prompt surgical exploration may be required.
- Unrecognized bowel injuries can be avoided by careful Veress needle and trocar placement and vigilance during dissection with electrocautery and ultrasonic shears.

REFERENCES

1. Kelling GU. Uber Oesophagoskopie, gastroskopie and zolioskopie. Munchene Medizinische Wochenschrift 1902; 49: 21–24.

2. Bishoff JT, Allaf ME, Kirkels W, Moore RG, Kavoussi LR, Schroder F. Laparoscopic bowel injury—incidence and clinical presentation. J Urol 1999; 161:887–890.

3. Chandler JG, Corson SL, Lawrence WW. Three spectra of laparoscopic entry access injuries. J Am Coll Surg 2001; 192:478–490.

4. El-Banna M, Abdel-Atty M, El-Meteini M, Aly S. Management of laparoscopic-related bowel injuries. Surg Endosc 2001; 14:779–782.

5. Birch DW, Park A, Shuhaibar H. Acute thermal injury to the canine jejunal free flap: electrocautery versus ultrasonic dissection. Am Surg 1997; 65:334–337.

6. Wang CW, Lee CL, Soong YK. Bowel injury by the suction irrigator during operative laparoscopy. J Am Assoc Gynecol Laparosc 1995; 2:353–354.

7. Chapron C, Querleu D, Bruhat MA, Madelenat P, Fernandez H, Pierre F, Dubuisson JB. Surgical complication of diagnostic and operative gynaecological laparoscopy: a series of 29,966 cases. Hum Reprod 1998; 13:867–872.

8. Bhoyrul S, Vierra MA, Nezhat CR, Krummel TM, Way LW. Trocar injuries in laparoscopic surgery. J Am Coll Surg 2001; 192:677–683.

9. Silen W. Copes Early Diagnosis of the Acute Abdomen. 19th ed. New York: Oxford University Press Inc., 1996:265–273.

10. Schwartz, Shires, Spencer. Principles of Surgery. 5th ed. New York: McGraw-Hill Book Company, 1989:1464–1469.

11. Li TC, Saravelos H, Richmond M, Cooke ID. Complications of laparoscopic pelvic surgery: recognition, management and prevention. Hum Reprod Update 1997; 3:505–515.

12. Almeida OD Jr, Val-Gallas JM. Small trocar perforation of the small bowel: a case report. JSLS 1998; 2:289–290.

13. Schäfer M, Lauper M, Krähenbühl L. Trocar and Veress needle injuries during laparoscopy. Surg Endosc 2001; 15: 275–280.

14. Thompson BH, Wheeless CR. Gastrointestinal complications of laparoscopic sterilization. Obstet Gynecol 1973; 41:669–676.

15. Ostrzenski A. Laparoscopic intestinal injury: a review and case presentation. J Natl Med Assoc 2001; 93:440–443.

16. Cruikshank AM, Fraser WD, Burns HJG, Van Damme J, Shenkin A. Response of serum interlukin-6 in patients undergoing surgery of varying severity. Clin Sci 1990; 79:161–165.

17. Kushner I, Ganapathi M, Schultz D. The acute phase response is mediated by heterogenous mechanisms. Ann New York Acad Sci 1989; 557:19–30.

18. Heinrich PC, Castell JV, Andus T. Interleukin-6 and the acute phase response. Biochem J 1990; 265:621–636.

19. Jakeways MS, Mitchell V, Hashim IA et al. Metabolic and inflammatory responses after open or laparoscopic cholecystectomy. Br J Surg 1994; 81:127–131.

20. Kloosterman T, von Blomberg BM, Borgstein P, Cuesta MA, Scheper RJ, Meijer S. Unimpaired immune functions after laparoscopic cholecystectomy. Surgery 1994; 115:424–428.

21. Joris J, Cigarini I, Legrand M, Jacquet N, De Groote D, Franchimont P, Lamy M. Metabolic and respiratory changes after cholecystectomy performed via laparotomy or laparoscopy. Br J Anaesth 1992; 69:341–345.

22. Mealy K, Gallagher H, Barry M, Lennon F, Traynor O, Hyland J. Physiological and metabolic responses to open and laparoscopic cholecystectomy. Br J Surg 1992; 79:1061–1064.

23. McMahon AJ, O'Dwyer PJ, Cruikshank A, McMillan D, Lowe G, Rumley A, O'Reilly D, Baxter JN. Metabolic changes after laparoscopic and minilaparoscopic cholecystectomy: a randomized trial. Br J Surg 1993; 80:641.

24. Harmon GD, Senagore AJ, Kilbride MJ, Warzynski MJ. Interleukin-6 response to laparoscopic and open colectomy. Dis Colon Rectum 1994; 37:754–759.

25. Cadeddu JA, Regan F, Kavoussi LR, Moore RG. The role of computerized tomography in the evaluation of complications after laparoscopic urological surgery. J Urol Oct 1997; 158: 1349–1352.

26. Reich H. Laparoscopic bowel injury. Surg Laparosc Endosc 1992; 2:74–78.

27. Nezhat C, Nezhat F, Ambroze W, Pennington E. Laparoscopic repair of small bowel and colon: a report of 26 cases. Surg Endosc 1993; 7:88–89.

28. Palmer R. Safety in laparoscopy. J Reprod Med 1974; 13:1–5.

29. Audebert AJ, Gomel, V. Role of microlaparoscopy in the diagnosis of peritoneal and visceral adhesions and in the prevention of bowel injury associated with blind trocar insertion. Fert Sterility 2000; 73:631–635.

30. Saye WB, Miller W, Hertzmann P. Electrosurgery thermal injury: myth or misconception. Surg Laparosc Endosc 1991; 4:223–228.

31. Soderstrom RM, Levinson C, Levy B. Complications of operative laparoscopy. In: Soderstrom RM, ed. Operative Laparscopy. New York: Raven Press, 1993:187–197.

32. Grosskinsky CM, Hulka JE. Unipolar electrosurgery in operative laparoscopy. Capacitance as a potential source of injury. J Reprod Med 1995; 40:549.

33. Tucker RD, Voyles CR, Silvis SE. Capacitive coupled stray currents during laparoscopic and endoscopic electrosurgical procedures. Biomed Instrum Technol 1992; 26:303–311.

34. Awwad JT, Isaacson K. The harmonic scalpel: an intraoperative complication. Obstet Gynecol 1996; 88:718–719.

6

Gallbladder, Pancreas and Splenic Injuries

JON VARKARAKIS
Second Department of Urology,
University of Athens, Athens, Greece

THOMAS JARRETT
Division of Urology,
Johns Hopkins Medical Institutions,
Baltimore, Maryland, U.S.A.

SANJAY RAMAKUMAR
University of Arizona Health Sciences
Center, Tucson, Arizona, U.S.A.

GALLBLADDER INJURIES

Gallbladder removal is one of the most commonly performed laparoscopic procedures and can occasionally be done in the same setting with a right laparoscopic nephrectomy or adrenalectomy. Accidental injury of this organ during right-sided urologic surgery may occur, as with any other organ. Gallbladder injuries, while very rare during urologic surgery, may occur during retraction of the liver and abdominal entry of laparoscopic instruments. If there is a laceration or puncture injury to the body of the gallbladder with leakage of bile, general surgery should be consulted for laparoscopic cholecystectomy. Superficial cautery burns to the wall of the gallbladder can be managed conservatively with placement of a closed suction drain in the gallbladder fossa and observation.

At the Johns Hopkins Hospital from a total of 717 laparoscopic procedures for upper urinary tract pathology, two gallbladder injuries occurred during 236 right-sided procedures (0.8%). One thermal injury and one tear after a difficult upper renal pole dissection lead to two unplanned cholecystectomies. On the other hand, elective removal of this organ at the time of urologic surgery was performed in seven (2.9%) patients. Operative times were 287.5 vs. 214.2 min for the inadvertent and the elective removal group, respectively. Operative times depended on the primary urologic procedure performed and not whether the cholecystectomy was planned or not. Time required for gallbladder removal was similar in both groups. No postoperative complications occurred in the accidental injury group. On the contrary, a postoperative bilious leak occurred in the elective removal group, which required TPN, drainage under CT guidance, and common bile duct stenting during ERCP, prolonging the patient's hospitalization significantly. Length of hospitalization was 5 vs. 6.4 days for the two groups, respectively. Once an injury is detected, removal of the gallbladder can be easily performed, but proper technique is required since a complication can occur even in selected planned cases.

PANCREATIC INJURIES

Intentional laparoscopic pancreatic resection for pancreatic diseases has been reported in the general surgery literature (1,2), but transection of this organ during urologic surgery is rare. If pancreatic injury is unrecognized, postoperative complications such as acute pancreatitis, pancreatic leakage, and pancreatic fistula can occur. Because of the severity of these complications, pancreatic injuries are usually presented separately in large series of laparoscopic urologic surgery and occur in about 0.2% of cases (3,4).

At the Johns Hopkins Hospital from a total of 717 laparoscopic procedures for upper urinary tract pathology, four pancreatic injuries occurred during 481 left-sided procedures (0.8%). Injuries occurred during difficult dissections for renal cell carcinoma (2), pheochromocytoma (1), and a mature cystic teratoma of the adrenal (1). Mean estimated blood loss was 237.5 mL and mean operating time was 215 min. In only one case, the pancreatic injury was recognized intraoperatively, but was considered small with no duct involvement and no further management other than drain placement was necessary. All other injuries were not recognized intraoperatively. In two patients, acute pancreatitis developed postoperatively resulting in a pancreaticocutaneous fistula in one. Conservative management with TPN was necessary in these patients, while multiple CT-guided drainage of the recurring pancreatic collection was necessary in one patient. In one case, pancreatic tissue had been resected with the endovascular stapler and the only evidence of injury was the existence of pancreatic tissue in the pathologic specimen.

No patient died although the hospital stay in one was significantly prolonged (mean hospital stay was 18 days, range 4–57 days). Only three patients had two Ranson criteria present, fact confirming the low severity of injuries in our small series of patients.

Injuries of the pancreatic tail are rare, but may occur during difficult dissection on left-sided procedures. Usually, these injuries can be missed intraoperatively. The clinical presentation of these injuries span between the two extremes; from an incidental finding of pancreatic tissue in the pathological specimen to a prolonged postoperative course requiring multiple procedures. Conservative measures and drainage are usually enough in the majority of cases since these are of low to medium severity.

Splenic Injuries

Splenectomy complicating left open nephrectomy has an incidence as high as 10%. The mechanisms of splenic injury can occur similarly in laparoscopic surgery, especially with large tumors of the upper pole of the left kidney. Published laparoscopic series report a splenectomy rate of 0.5% (3). Several methods may lessen the risk of splenic injury (5). When practical, a retroperitoneal approach significantly reduces splenic injury. Multiple studies have recognized that traction on the splenic ligaments is the leading cause of injury. Adequate incision of the lieno-colic, lieno-renal, and lieno-omental bands will allow for passive reflection of the pancreas and spleen. Splenorrhaphy is possible with minor injury with fibrin sealant reported to be successful (6). In cases of severe blood loss, coagulopathy, or patient instability, splenectomy is preferred with general surgery consultation as required.

KEY POINTS

- Laceration or puncture injury to the gallbladder should be treated with cholecystectomy.
- Minor superficial gallbladder burns should be monitored with closed suction drainage.
- Conservative measures will treat the majority of pancreatic injuries.
- Adequate incision of splenic ligaments can reduce the risk of injury during left nephrectomy.

REFERENCES

1. Minni F, Marrano N, Pasquali R. Laparoscopic body-tail pancreatic resection for insulinoma. Surg Endosc 2003; 17:159–160.

2. Ueno T, Oka M, Nishihara K, Yamamoto K, Nakamura M, Yahara N, Adachi T. Laparoscopic distal pancreatectomy with preservation of the spleen. Surg Laparosc Endosc Percutan Tech 1999; 9:290–293.

3. Fahlenkamp D, Rassweiler J, Fornara P, Frede T, Loening SA. Complications of laparoscopic procedures in urology: experience with 2,407 procedures at 4 German centers. Urology 1999; 162:765–770.

4. Vallancien G, Cathelineau X, Baumert H, Doublet JD, Guillonneau B. Complications of transperitoneal laparoscopic surgery in urology: review of 1,311 procedures at a single center. Urology 2002; 168:23–26.

5. Cooper CS, Cohen MB, Donovan JF. Splenectomy complicating left nephrectomy. J Urol 1996; 155:30–36.

6. Canby-Hagino ED, Morey AF, Jatoi I, Perahia B, Bishoff JT. Fibrin sealant treatment of splenic injury during open and laparoscopic left radical nephrectomy. J Urol 2000; 164:2004–2005.

7

Liver Injury During Urologic Laparoscopy

KENNETH OGAN and JEFFREY A. CADEDDU

The Clinical Center for Minimally Invasive
Urologic Cancer Treatment, Department of
Urology, University of Texas, Southwestern
Medical Center at Dallas, Dallas, Texas, U.S.A.

INTRODUCTION

The liver is one of the largest solid organs in the body, making up approximately one-fiftieth of the total body weight. The intraperitoneal lower border of the liver extends well below the costal margin on the right side. It is made up of two lobes separated by a line drawn from the IVC to the gallbladder fossa, and has a dual blood supply from the hepatic artery and portal vein. Due to its large size and intraabdominal location it is at risk for injury during transperitoneal laparoscopic operations. The majority of injuries occur either during

73

needle/trocar insertion or from retraction of the liver during right kidney or adrenal surgery. Fortunately, the majority of injuries to the liver encountered during urologic laparoscopy is minor and can be managed laparoscopically. However, urologists should have a low threshold for conversion to an open procedure if an extensive injury occurs.

ABDOMINAL ACCESS AND LIVER RETRACTION INJURIES

A small percentage of laparoscopic vascular and organ injuries occur during initial abdominal access with the Veress needle or from initial trocar entry. Fortunately, the liver is rarely involved. A review from four German centers that performed 2407 urologic laparoscopic cases reported an overall complication rate of 4.4% (1). The most common injuries were to vascular structures (1.7%) and to the viscera (1.1%). Of these, 0.2% occurred during initial abdominal cavity access, with liver injury not specifically mentioned. In a prospective review by Schafer et al. (2) of laparoscopic procedures performed by the Swiss Association for Laparoscopic and Thoracoscopic Surgery between 1995 and 1997, there were 22 trocar and four needle injuries (incidence = 0.18%). The small bowel was the single most affected organ (six cases), followed by the large bowel and the liver (three cases each). Of the 23 injuries noted intraoperatively, only five (21.7%) could be managed laparoscopically, with the balance requiring open conversion and repair. In an effort to minimize the incidence of access-related injuries, open trocar placement (Hasson technique) has been advocated. However, even with this technique, iatrogenic injury may occur (3). Also, the recent description of a radially expanding trocar system (VersStep Access System, US Surgical Corporation, Norwalk, CT) has also been reported to decrease access-related complications. Shekarriz et al. (4) recently used these trocars in 62 upper tract urologic laparoscopic cases (24 with prior abdominal surgery) without any access-related complications.

Liver retraction is commonly required when performing procedures on the right kidney and adrenal gland. Unfortunately, improper retraction or inadvertent retractor movements can result in liver laceration, though its frequency is unreported. Prior to liver manipulation, all adhesions to the peritoneum or surrounding structures must be taken down to prevent tearing of the liver capsule with retraction. We tend to favor a 3 mm locking grasper that is placed across and under the edge of the liver from medial to lateral. This is held in place by locking onto the peritoneum of the right abdominal wall (Fig. 1). Since it is placed across the liver, there is minimal opportunity for liver injury even when the liver is outside the laparoscope's field of view. A fan retractor or S-shaped retractor can also be placed under the liver for retraction but their larger profile may interfere with the intended dissection. Pautler et al. (5) have developed an articulating retractor holder that is secured to the operating table for retraction of the liver or spleen during kidney and adrenal procedures. As without technique, not only does a mechanical holder free the assistant surgeon from holding a retractor, it will not move or fatigue. Therefore, a blunt liver retractor that does not impair dissection, and will not change

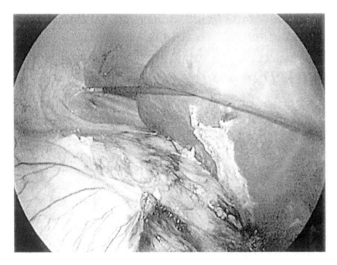

Figure 1 Three millimeter locking grasper retracting the liver to expose the upper pole of the right kidney.

position inadvertently during the procedure should help prevent liver injuries secondary to retraction.

KEYS TO DIAGNOSIS

If there is a substantial injury to the liver during laparoscopic surgery it will become evident quickly. After insertion of the Veress needle into the right upper quadrant of the abdomen, aspiration of blood or bile is indicative of a hepatic or gall bladder injury. Should this occur, the abdomen is entered at another location while leaving the Veress needle in place. Once in the abdomen, laparoscopic inspection of the liver injury can easily be done by following the path of the Veress needle.

Injuries to the liver during trocar placement, liver retraction, or high retroperitoneal dissection are usually obvious as soon as they occur, and are manifested by continuous hemorrhage. Small superficial lacerations may not be as obvious and, therefore, the liver should always be systematically evaluated under a low intraabdominal pressure (5 mmHg) at the termination of the case. The low pressure may unmask parenchymal bleeding that can then be managed appropriately. Inadvertent lacerations of the gallbladder can usually be seen by the accumulation of bile in the gallbladder fossa.

MANAGEMENT STRATEGIES

The majority of injuries to the liver are minor, consisting of a small laceration or puncture injury. If the bleeding is minimal and not disrupting the surgical dissection, it should be left alone as it may stop spontaneously. Persistent bleeding requires cauterization with either electrocautery (at high power settings) or the argon beam coagulator. Following this maneuver, oxidized cellulose may be placed over the site and welded to the surface of the liver with either the electrocautery or argon beam electrocoagulator. In an effort to prevent delayed hemorrhage or assist with persistent bleeding, fibrin glue can be applied over the entire repair. Ishitani et al. (6)

found that fibrin glue could be accurately applied to the base of liver injuries using laparoscopic guidance with rapid control of hepatic bleeding. For bleeding after laparoscopic liver biopsy, Dagnini et al. (7) advocate the use of a fibrin sponge to plug the biopsy defect. This should also be considered for significant lacerations.

Moderate hemorrhage associated with parenchymal lacerations usually will not respond to electrocautery or the aforementioned hemostatic agents. In these cases, repair is usually accomplished with the use of parenchymal compression sutures. If indicated, consultation with a laparoscopic general surgeon is recommended as this is not easily performed laparoscopically and may prompt open conversion. In an effort to increase visualization and decrease blood loss, the general surgeon can perform the Pringle maneuver (clamping the porta hepatis). This maneuver has been shown to facilitate laparoscopic wedge resections and partial hepatic lobectomies (8). Concerns of hemodynamic instability secondary to portal triad occlusion and pneumoperitoneum have been disproved (9).

For those patients who suffer severe bleeding from the liver because of laceration of a major hepatic vessel, a deep or large parenchymal laceration, or the presence of a coagulapathy, the only means of controlling the hemorrhage may be temporary pack tamponade. This technique has only been described in open surgery, and in the face of such major bleeding, general surgery assistance and conversion to an open procedure is mandatory. This would involve packing the perihepatic region with multiple lap sponges until the bleeding stops and then returning for pack removal 24–96 hr later when the patient is stable. A treatment algorithm for laparoscopic liver injury is illustrated in Figure 2.

Delayed hepatic bleeding is an extremely rare event, which has been reported following percutaneous liver biopsies, though not after urologic laparoscopic procedures. Nevertheless, awareness that this could occur is mandatory. In a review of the world literature, Reichert et al. (10) in 1983 reported only 15 cases of delayed hemorrhage following

Degree of Liver Bleeding

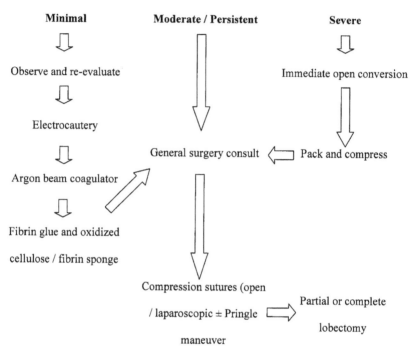

Figure 2   Treatment algorithm for laparoscopic liver injury.

liver biopsy that occurred between 36 hr and 18 days post biopsy. The etiology was usually secondary to pseudoaneurysm formation and patient presentation varied from no symptoms to hemobilia and massive fatal hemorrhage. Doppler ultrasound and contrast CT imaging was used for diagnosis, with selective visceral arteriography reserved for patients with negative initial studies and a high index of suspicion. First-line treatment for delayed hepatic bleeding should entail selective embolization of the responsible hepatic artery branch or pseudoaneurysm. This has a success rate of 97% as reported by Tsai et al. (11) for pseudoaneurysms postcholecystectomy. If embolization fails, hepatic lobectomy and open exploration are required.

PREVENTION TECHNIQUES

Laparoscopic liver injuries may be difficult to manage; thus, meticulous care to avoid them is necessary. Most injuries usually occur during laparoscopic access, liver retraction or when dissecting the upper pole of the right kidney and adrenal gland. Not placing the Veress needle in the right upper quadrant will avoid many liver injuries. However, in patients with hepatomegaly, the liver edge may extend across the midline and below the umbilicus. Therefore, it is always prudent to assess the position of the liver on the preoperative radiographic images prior to Veress needle placement. Once within the abdomen, injury from trocar placement is less likely as these should always be placed under direct laparoscopic visualization.

There are a number of different retractors and techniques available for liver retraction during laparoscopic dissection of the right kidney and adrenal. We tend to favor a 3 mm locking grasper, which is placed through a 3 mm port just below the costal margin 1–2 cm to the left of the midline. The instrument is then swept underneath the falciform ligament and edge of the liver. The liver is elevated appropriately and the peritoneum of the right abdominal wall is grasped to lock the instrument in place (self-retaining). The key to avoiding liver injury during this maneuver is to extend the grasper under the entire right lobe of the liver so that the tip of the grasper does not puncture the liver parenchyma. The alternative is the commercial fan-shaped retractors placed through a separate lateral port (5 or 10 mm). Again, the key to avoid puncture injuries of the liver is to use a broad contact surface.

KEY POINTS

- Liver injury is rare during urologic laparoscopy.
- Injury can occur during access, liver retraction, and kidney/adrenal dissection.
- Minor injuries are easily controlled with electrocautery, argon beam coagulation, and oxidized cellulose.

- Moderate injuries require intracorporeal suturing and should be done in conjunction with a laparoscopic general surgeon.
- Severe injuries mandate immediate open conversion.
- Liver injuries can be prevented by controlled abdominal access away from the liver and broad-based laparoscopic liver retractors.

REFERENCES

1. Fahlenkamp D, Rassweiler J, Fornara P, Frede T, Loening SA. Complications of laparoscopic procedures in urology: experience with 2,407 procedures at 4 German centers. J Urol 1999; 162:765–770; discussion 770–771.

2. Schafer M, Lauper M, Krahenbuhl L. Trocar and Veress needle injuries during laparoscopy. Surg Endosc 2001; 15:275–280.

3. Bonjer HJ, Hazebroek EJ, Kazemier G, Giuffrida MC, Meijer WS, Lange JF. Open versus closed establishment of pneumoperitoneum in laparoscopic surgery. Br J Surg 1997; 84: 599–602.

4. Shekarriz B, Gholami SS, Rudnick DM, Duh QY, Stoller ML. Radially expanding laparoscopic access for renal/adrenal surgery. Urology 2001; 58:683–687.

5. Pautler SE, McWilliams GW, Harrington FS, Walther MM. An articulating retractor holder to facilitate laparoscopic adrenalectomy and nephrectomy. J Urol 2001; 166:198–199.

6. Ishitani MB, McGahren ED, Sibley DA, Spotnitz WD, Rodgers BM. Laparoscopically applied fibrin glue in experimental liver trauma. J Pediatr Surg 1989; 24:867–871.

7. Dagnini G, Caldironi MW, Marin G, Patella M. Fibrin sponge plugging of hemorrhage from laparoscopic biopsy. Gastrointest Endosc 1985; 31:35–36.

8. Abdel-Atty MY, Farges O, Jagot P, Belghiti J. Laparoscopy extends the indications for liver resection in patients with cirrhosis. Br J Surg 1999; 86:1397–1400.

9. Decailliot F, Cherqui D, Leroux B, Lanteri-Minet M, Ben Said S, Husson E, et al. Effects of portal triad clamping on haemo-

dynamic conditions during laparoscopic liver resection. Br J Anaesth 2001; 87:493–496.

10. Reichert CM, Weisenthal LM, Klein HG. Delayed hemorrhage after percutaneous liver biopsy. J Clin Gastroenterol 1983; 5:263–266.

11. Garby KB, King TS, Tsai FY. Recurrence of pseudoaneurysm after successful embolization. J Endovasc Surg 1997; 4: 385–388.

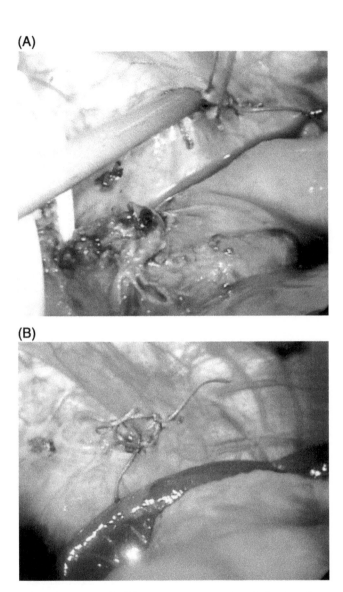

Figure 8.1 (A) Pleurotomy sustained during laparoscopic donor nephrectomy is closed with interrupted vicryl sutures. Air is evacuated from the pleural cavity prior to securing final stitches using the laparoscopic suction device through the pleurotomy. (B) Final stitches are secured, closing the pleurotomy.

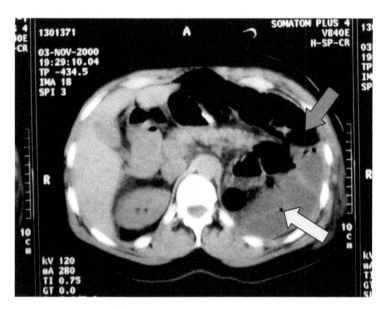

Figure 11.1 CT imaging of an internal hernia after left laparoscopic radical nephrectomy. Dilated small bowel (yellow arrow) is seen posterior to the descending colon (red arrow).

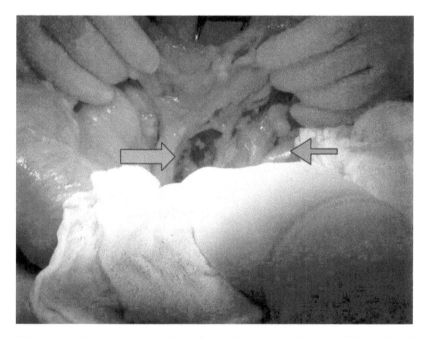

Figure 11.2 Intraoperative photo demonstrating small bowel (red arrow) reduced from the defect in the descending colon mesentery (green arrow). Small bowel resection was not necessary.

8

Pleural Injury During Laparoscopic Renal Surgery

JOSEPH J. DEL PIZZO

James Buchanan Brady Urological Foundation,
The New York-Presbyterian Hospital,
University Hospital of Cornell,
New York, New York, U.S.A.

INTRODUCTION

With its clearly defined advantages over traditional open surgery, laparoscopy has gained global popularity and widespread
use in the treatment of surgical pathological conditions in a
wide variety of specialties. Surveys of complications from
laparoscopy have been reported for abdominal and pelvic procedures (1). Injury to the diaphragm is an uncommon yet
acknowledged complication of laparoscopic surgery, and one
with potentially disastrous sequelae, especially if not recognized
intraoperatively.

In the field of urology, laparoscopic renal surgery is becoming part of the clinical armamentarium of more and more surgeons. As surgeons learn this operation, they must become familiar with the variety of potential complications that exist. This includes the potential for injury to the pleura, a complication commonly seen with open surgical approaches but rarely during laparoscopic renal surgery. In addition, the laparoscopist must learn surgical techniques for avoidance, recognition, and management of a pleural injury and its sequelae, including pneumothorax.

INTRAOPERATIVE RECOGNITION

Inadvertent entry into the pleural space during open flank surgery is typically recognized intraoperatively and repaired without sequela. Recognition of a pleural injury during laparoscopic renal surgery may be more subtle and difficult to identify, especially to the relatively inexperienced laparoscopist. Unlike its open counterpart, laparoscopic renal surgery entails the use of carbon dioxide insufflation of the peritoneal or retroperitoneal space under pressure. This insufflated gas can enter the thoracic cavity through small, difficult to recognize diaphragmatic tears, leading to sudden collapse of the ipsilateral lung. The resulting pneumothorax may lead to sudden changes in the intraoperative cardiopulmonary status of the patient. An undiagnosed injury has the potential for being a disastrous complication. Therefore, intraoperative recognition and management of a pleural injury is a crucial step in the learning curve for laparoscopic renal surgery.

Iatrogenic injury to the pleura during laparoscopic surgery has been attributed to iatrogenic injury to the diaphragm, biopsy of a metastatic implant on the diaphragm, congenital defects of the diaphragm, pneumomediastinum, and postoperative vomiting (1,2). Most reports detailing pleural injury during laparoscopic renal surgery have been limited to case reports and technical considerations (3–7). Recently, our institution reported on a retrospective review of a large, multiinstitutional series of laparoscopic renal cases, looking at the incidence of pleural injury, as well as the mechanism of injury, intraoperative recognition, and management (8).

In this series, all cases where an intraoperative injury to the pleura occurred during dissection of the kidney were performed via an intraperitoneal approach. In six of these eight cases, a recognized pleurotomy was made. This included injury during splenic mobilization to expose the upper pole of the kidney on the left side (two cases), liver mobilization to expose the upper pole on the right side (two cases), mobilization of a large tumor on the upper pole of the right kidney (one case), and during mobilization of the ascending colon to expose the right kidney (one case). Of these cases, three were associated with injury from monopolar electrocautery, and three with injury from the harmonic scalpel.

In the other two cases, no frank injury in the diaphragm or pleura was recognized, but the surgeon noted the diaphragm billowing down into the surgical field. One case involved dissection of a large right mid pole renal tumor off of the diaphragm, the other involved dissection of a large left upper pole renal cyst off of the diaphragm. In both instances, close inspection of the area where the lesion was adjacent to the diaphragm revealed a small monopolar cautery burn. Despite the absence of a clearly defined pleurotomy and any respiratory findings, a diaphragmatic injury was strongly suspected. Anesthesia reported no decrease in breath sounds, acute hypercarbia, or change in inspiratory pressures in these cases.

In two cases, injury to the diaphragm was due to inadvertent placement of a trocar through the pleural cavity. Both cases involved laparoscopic extirpative renal surgery through a posterior retroperitoneal approach. In each case, a trocar was placed under direct vision along the costal margin too close to the ribs and subsequently through the pleura. Soon after trocar placement, the anesthesiologist noted carbon dioxide retention, hemodynamic instability, and no breath sounds on the left side of the chest. Release of pneumoretroperitoneum resulted in prompt resolution of all of these signs consistent with a tension pneumothorax.

MANAGEMENT

The review of our series showed that in the six cases, where a definitive pleurotomy was recognized by the surgeon, the defect was repaired laparoscopically. Anesthesia was consulted at the time of injury to monitor respiratory sounds on both sides and airway pressures. Although breath sounds became diminished on the side of injury, and airway pressures became moderately elevated, each patient remained hemodynamically stable with no acute hypercarbia. In this instance, the pneumoperitoneum is lowered from 15–20 mmHg to 10 mmHg, and the nephrectomy completed with close monitoring of the patient's hemodynamic and respiratory status. After the specimen was removed, the abdomen was reinsufflated and the pleurotomy addressed with the kidney specimen no longer in the surgeon's way.

The pleural cavity can be inspected with the laparoscope, ensuring no direct pulmonary injury. Using the laparoscopic automated suturing device (Endostitch, US Surgical, Norwalk, CT) or laparoscopic needle drivers with a free needle and suture, the diaphragmatic injury and pleurotomy is reapproximated using four interrupted figures of eight, 2-0 vicryl sutures. Prior to the final closure, air is evacuated from the pleural cavity by placing the laparoscopic suction device through the defect (Fig. 1A), and the stitches are secured (Fig. 1B). Alternatively, the patient can be given a large inspiratory breath prior to securing the stitches. This was performed in two cases. The surgeon then used a 6 French central line, modified by cutting extra side holes and placed it into the sixth intercostals space anteriorly using a Seldinger technique. Residual air was then aspirated from the pleural space. Postoperative chest x-rays showed full expansion of the lung in all but one case, where a residual pneumothorax was seen. This was managed with postoperative tube thoracostomy. The tube was removed on postoperative day 2, and the patient was discharged home the next day. No long-term sequelae were noted in any patient.

Two cases involved diaphragmatic injuries suspected when the surgeon noted billowing of the diaphragm into the surgical field as a large lesion was being dissected off of the diaphragm. This is classically referred to as the "floppy

(A)

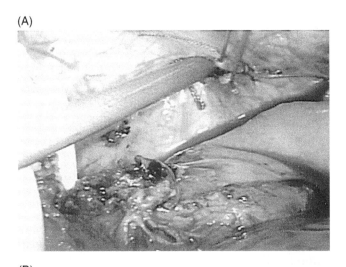

(B)

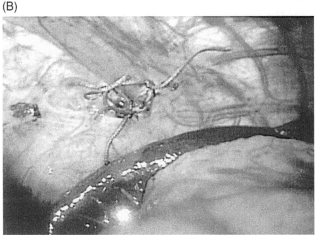

Figure 1 (A) Pleurotomy sustained during laparoscopic donor nephrectomy is closed with interrupted vicryl sutures. Air is evacuated from the pleural cavity prior to securing final stitches using the laparoscopic suction device through the pleurotomy. (B) Final stitches are secured, closing the pleurotomy. (*See color insert*)

diaphragm" sign, and reflects the loss of negative pressure within the diaphragm. In each case, despite the absence of respiratory findings, there was strong clinical suspicion of a diaphragmatic injury. A small cautery burn was discovered on the diaphragm in the area of renal dissection. In both cases, the intraabdominal pressure was reduced to 10 mmHg and an additional posterior trocar was placed to aid with cephalad retraction of the "floppy" diaphragm. Laparoscopic sutures were used to oversew the area where the cautery burn was seen on the diaphragm. After this was completed, the billowing of the diaphragm stopped, and the cases were completed. Prior to extubation, a chest x-ray was obtained, which showed a complete pneumothorax in one case, which was evacuated using the previously described modified 6 French central line. The second patient was found to have no residual pneumothorax. No long-term sequelae were noted in any patient.

Our two cases involving placement of trocars into the pleural cavity during retroperitoneoscopic nephrectomy were ultimately managed with placement of a 24 French chest tube. In one case, the trocar was placed at the beginning of the case, and the patient showed increased airway pressures soon afterwards, necessitating chest tube placement before the procedure could be completed. In the second case, the trocar was placed at the end of the case prior to removal of a partial nephrectomy specimen. Using a pressure of 10 mmHg, the surgeon was able to finish the case without difficulty before proceeding with tube thoracostomy. Each patient was treated with chest tube decompression for 48 hr. Follow-up chest films showed no residual pneumothorax. Both patients recovered without complication.

DISCUSSION

Injury to the diaphragm is an uncommon yet recognized complication of several laparoscopic procedures (1,9,10). Often, proper transabdominal exposure for both extirpative and donor nephrectomy involves wide mobilization of intraabdominal organs including the liver, spleen, pancreas, and colon. In addition, large upper or mid-pole renal lesions often must be carefully dissected away from the body wall. Tears of the parietal pleura may then allow passage of intraabdominal CO_2 under pressure into the pleural cavity and lead to pneumothorax.

Early recognition of a diaphragmatic injury is critical for prompt management and avoidance of potentially dangerous sequelae, including pneumothorax, pneumomediastinum, hypercarbia, and subcutaneous emphysema. In our series, the majority of injuries occurred from surgical dissection close to the diaphragm, either during mobilization of intraabdominal structures for exposure of the kidney, or during dissection of large mass structures off of the diaphragm. These injuries were recognized immediately by the experienced laparoscopic surgeon, and managed intraoperatively.

The timing of management of the injury is correlated with the clinical condition of the patient. The anesthesiologist is a critical component of the decision-making process for repair of the injury. The anesthesiologist should be alerted immediately of the injury in order to monitor changes in the patient's cardiopulmonary status, as diffusion of carbon dioxide into the pleural cavity often will result in a decrease in oxygen saturation, an increase in airway pressures, an increase in end-tidal CO_2, decrease in breath sounds, and hemodynamic instability (3). These are important parameters for the laparoscopic surgeon to understand, as a small injury to the pleura may go unrecognized intraoperatively.

Once recognized, if the patient is stable, the procedure can continue and the injury can be addressed at the end of the case. Often times, we found that the kidney, especially if a large tumor was present or other intraabdominal organs obstructed the injury from the surgeon's view, hindered immediate repair. Once the case is completed and the specimen removed, there is more room for the surgeon to safely repair the injury. A pleurotomy can be oversewn using a variety of laparoscopic suturing devices. Before securing the stitches, air is evacuated from the pleural cavity using either a suction device, a modified central line, or by having the anesthesiologist give the patient a large inspiratory breath. With experience, most diaphragmatic injuries can be repaired promptly and without the need for tube thoracostomy.

The surgeon may be alerted to an unrecognized injury by the "floppy diaphragm" sign, whereby the diaphragm billows inferiorly with any degree of desufflation of the abdomen, thus reflecting the loss of negative pressure within the diaphragm (4). In two cases in this series, there was strong clinical suspicion of a diaphragmatic injury based upon this sign despite the absence of respiratory findings or recognized pleurotomy. We addressed the potential injury in order to improve our anatomic exposure, which was obscured by the billowing diaphragm. One patient had a residual pneumothorax after desufflation of the abdomen that required air evacuation. There are reports that intervention is not necessary for this finding in a stable patient as the pneumothorax typically resolves upon desufflation of the pneumoperitoneum (4). It is nonetheless important for the novice laparoscopic surgeon to be aware of this objective finding to raise suspicion of an unrecognized diaphragmatic injury. In addition, suspicion should be higher on the right side, as an asymptomatic injury may go unrecognized since the liver may prevent billowing of the diaphragm.

The remaining two cases of pleural injury were sustained by inadvertent placement of a trocar into the pleural space during a laparoscopic retroperitoneal approach. Prevention comes from experience and careful attention to detail. Management of these cases centered upon prompt recognition and close patient monitoring. Due to some degree of hemodynamic instability and pulmonary compromise, tube thoracostomy was performed, and this is always a safe way to manage a diaphragmatic injury if repair cannot be done safely.

The potential for diaphragmatic injury during laparoscopic renal surgery should be a part of the surgeon's approach to each case, especially those where an injury may be more likely, such as patients with large upper or mid renal lesions or inflammatory cysts. Limited use of monopolar electrocautery in areas where visualization may be diminished due to these lesions may be a way to avoid injury to the pleura. In this series, several of the injuries were sustained later in the laparoscopic series. Therefore, even the experienced laparoscopic surgeon must remain keenly aware of the potential for pleural injury during select cases. Surgeons should have a low threshold for postoperative chest x-ray examination in these cases as injuries may go unrecognized intraoperatively if there are no intraoperative signs. A proper course of management after a pleural injury is seen or suspected poses a challenge for the laparoscopic surgeon, as it involves close monitoring of the patient's cardiopulmonary status, repair of the defect including evacuation of the air in the pleural space, and postoperative monitoring for evidence of a residual pneumothorax (5).

KEY POINTS

- Pleural injury is an uncommon but potentially serious complication of laparoscopic renal procedures.
- Use meticulous dissection when mobilizing the spleen, liver, colon and especially large upper or mid-pole renal lesions that may be in close proximity to the fibers of the diaphragm.
- Minimize use of cautery when dissecting lesions near the diaphragm.
- Maintain a high index of suspicion when the diaphragm is seen billowing down into the surgical field.
- Inform the anesthesiologist to closely monitor the patient's cardiopulmonary status.
- If the patient is stable, lower the pneumoperitoneum to 10 mmHg and finish the procedure before addressing the pleurotomy.
- Close the pleurotomy under direct vision, making sure to evacuate the air from the pleural cavity.
- Maintain a low threshold for tube thoracostomy should the patient become unstable after a diaphragmatic injury is sustained.

REFERENCES

1. Bishoff J, Kirkels W, Moore R, Kavoussi L, Schroder F. Laparoscopic bowel injury: incidence and unique clinical presentation. J Urol 1999; 161:887–890.

2. Reid DB, Winning T, Bell G. Pneumothorax during laparoscopic dissection of the diaphragmatic hiatus. Br J Surg 1993; 80:670–672.

3. Loffer ED, Pent D. Indications, contraindications, and complications of laparoscopy. Obstet Gynecol Surg 1975; 30:407–419.

4. Dunnick NR, Ozols RF, Long JA. Radiographic contribution to diagnosis and treatment of complications from peritoneoscopy. Gastrointest Radiol 1981; 6:69–79.

5. Joris JL, Chiche JD, Lamy ML. Pneumothorax during laparoscopic fundoplication: diagnosis and treatment with positive end-expiratory pressure. Anesth Analg 1995; 81:993–995.

6. Voyles CR, Madden B. The "floppy diaphragm" sign with laparoscopic-associated pneumothorax. JSLS 1998; 2:71–74.

7. Potter SR, Kavoussi LR, Jackman SV. Management of diaphragmatic injury during laparoscopic nephrectomy. J Urol 2001; 165:1203–1205.

8. Del Pizzo JJ, Jacobs SC, Bishoff JT, Kavoussi LR, Jarrett TJ. Pleural injury during laparoscopic renal surgery: early recognition and management. J Urol. 2003; 169(1):41–44.

9. Hedican SP, Wolf JS, Moon TD, Rayhill SC, Seifman BD, Nakada SY. Complications of hand-assisted laparoscopy in urologic surgery. J Urol 2002; 167(suppl):22–23.

10. Richard HM, Stancato-Pasik A, Salky BA. Pneumothorax and pneumomediastinum after laparoscopic surgery. Clin Imag 1997; 21:337.

9

Urinary Leak Complications of Laparoscopy

GEORGE K. CHOW

Department of Urology, Mayo Clinic,
Rochester, Minnesota, U.S.A.

INTRODUCTION

Fortunately, injury resulting in urinary leak is rare. The incidence of urinary tract injury with laparoscopic urology varies between 0.4% and 0.7% (1–3). It is as common or more common for the urologist to encounter laparoscopic urinary tract injury as a consultation from other services. Advanced gynecologic laparoscopy (hysterectomy, ovarian cystectomy, adnexectomy, endometriosis ablation) is associated with a urinary complication rate of 0.42–1.6% (4–7). Laparoscopic colorectal surgery is associated with a 0–2.0% risk of urinary tract injury (8–10). It is understandable that colorectal and gynecology surgery would be at risk given the fact that they share the same operative anatomic region as the urologist.

Injuries to the bladder and ureter are the most commonly reported urinary leak complications in the medical literature. Though the urethra and renal pelvis theoretically may be subject to injury during laparoscopy, this is usually a complication of reconstructive laparoscopic surgery such as laparoscopic pyeloplasty or urethrovesical anastomosis for laparoscopic prostatectomy.

URETERAL INJURIES

The likelihood and location of ureteral injury seem to correlate with the proximity of the ureter to the operative target. For example, in laparoscopic-assisted vaginal hysterectomy, the location of ureteral injury occurs where the ureter crosses close to the cervix adjacent to the cardinal ligament (11). Likewise, the ureter can be injured near the ovarian vessels in the infundibulopelvic ligament in adnexal surgery (11). In laparoscopic colorectal surgery, the risk of ureteral injury is increased with dissection carried too laterally from the rectum (10).

Mechanism of injury includes division, ligation, and cauterization. Interruption of the ureteral blood supply can cause necrosis. A necrotic ureter can leak or stricture. Division of the ureter is often recognized intraoperatively. In contrast, delayed recognition of injury is more common with ligation and cautery injuries.

Recognition

Unless one is dealing with an obvious ureteral division, intraoperative recognition of ureteral injuries requires high clinical suspicion of injury. Recognition of ureteral injury is facilitated by the intravenous administration of methylene blue. Other maneuvers that may help include the preoperative placement of a stent on high-risk cases.

Postoperatively, ureteral injury may present as fever, hematuria, or flank/abdominal pain. Peritonitis can be due to urinary ascites. A fistula can form to the surgical wound or vagina. If a surgical drain or urinary fistula is present, fluid can be sent for creatinine measurement. The drain fluid creatinine can then be compared to serum creatinine. A drain fluid creatinine that is very high compared to serum is consistent with urine.

If suspicion for an ureterovaginal fistula exists, a pad test with methylene blue can be used to confirm it. If uncertainty exists between the diagnoses of ureterovaginal and vesicovaginal fistula, a "double dye" pad test can be performed with oral Pyridium and vesical methylene blue with a clamped Foley catheter. Blue staining of a pad indicates a vesicovaginal fistula, orange suggests ureterovaginal fistula.

In the absence of drain fluid, radiographic evaluation with ultrasound or CT scan can identify urinoma or ascites. CT scan may be the most useful test in evaluating postoperative laparoscopic patients. Cadeddu and colleagues (3) determined that CT scans identified symptom-related diagnosis in 75% of patients evaluated postoperatively. Powsner and colleagues (12) advocate the usage of Tc-99m mercaptotriacetylglycine (MAG3) renal scan to identify urinary leak.

Management

Once a ureteral leak is confirmed, identification of the exact site of leak is critical. Retrograde pyelography can identify the exact site of ureteral extravasation. If a nephrostomy tube is present, an antegrade pyelogram can be equally efficacious.

Small ureteral injuries can be managed with ureteral stenting for 4–8 weeks. For urinary fistula, conservative management may be first attempted with stenting and/or proximal diversion with nephrostomy.

If complete avulsion of the ureter is identified or if conservative measures fail, surgical exploration and repair will be necessary. If delayed recognition occurs, an open exploration and repair would be advisable. The method of repair would depend on the level of injury. If a proximal or mid-ureteral injury is identified intraoperatively, a laparoscopic uretero-ureterostomy can be performed (Fig. 1). Laparoscopic ureteroneocystostomy, psoas hitch, or Boari flap can be per-

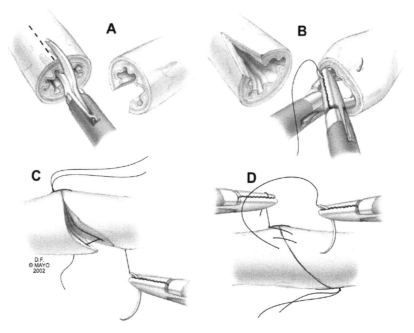

Figure 1 Laparoscopic uretero-ureterostomy. (A) After excising devitalized tissue, the ureteral ends are spatulated with endoscopic scissors. (B) An apical stitch using absorbable suture is placed at the 12 o'clock position of the distal ureteral end and placed into the proximal ureter at its corresponding 12 o'clock position. (C) After the 12 o'clock stitch is placed, a 6 o'clock stitch is placed in a similar fashion. (D) A running anastomosis is performed. A knot can be tied to the free end of the 6 o'clock knot.

formed for distal ureteral injuries. Laparoscopic uretero-ureterostomy or ureteroneocystostomy should only be attempted by a laparoscopist comfortable with intracorporeal suturing techniques.

Prevention

Several maneuvers can be performed to prevent ureteral injuries. In anticipation of probable urinary tract injury, a ureteral stent or ureteral catheter can be placed preoperatively. Also, initial identification of the ureter can be performed to avoid injury. In the absence of tactile feedback, lighted stents can also be used to help identify the ureter. Ureteral peristalsis can help confirm the identity of the ureter. For laparoscopic colectomy, Larach and Gallagher (10) recommend conversion to open surgery if the ureters are not identified.

BLADDER INJURIES

Bladder injuries can occur due to trocar placement, anatomic proximity of the bladder to the surgical site (laparoscopic Burch colposuspension), or due to factors complicating pelvic dissection (inflammatory mass, fibrosis). Trocar placement, though often maligned as a cause of bladder injury, is rarely associated with such injuries. In a French study of 103,852 laparoscopic surgery patients, trocar injuries accounted for only two bladder injuries (13).

Recognition

As with ureteral injuries, bladder injuries can present with fever, abdominal pain, and hematuria. Urinary ascites can present with ileus, abdominal distension, and increased peritoneal drain output. Vesicovaginal and vesicocutaneous fistulae can form. The pad test and "double dye" pad test described earlier can be used to evaluate for fistulae.

Radiographic evaluation consists of cystogram or CT cystogram. Having a lateral and postdrainage film are essential for accurate identification of bladder extravasation. The advantage of CT cystogram is increased sensitivity for evaluation of vesical fistulae.

Management

Intraoperative bladder injury can be repaired at time of surgery. Laparoscopic bladder repair can be performed with a two-layer closure with Vicryl suture. Extraperitoneal leaks can be managed conservatively with Foley catheter drainage for 7–10 days. If intraperitoneal leakage with urinary ascites is present, a formal open two- or three-layer repair is recommended.

Prevention

The most important preventive measure to take is to completely decompress the bladder with Foley catheter prior to trocar placement. Also, staying in the correct surgical plane is essential. If there is any question about bladder injury intraoperatively, methylene blue can be instilled via the Foley catheter.

RENAL PELVIC/COLLECTING SYSTEM INJURIES

There are few instances when the renal pelvis may be subject to injury during laparoscopic surgery. The renal pelvis and uretero–pelvic junction may leak urine after laparoscopic pyeloplasty. These injuries can present as flank pain, fever, and hematuria. The initial 100 laparoscopic pyeloplasties at Johns Hopkins incurred a 2% incidence of postoperative urine leak (14). CT scan is useful for evaluating these injuries. For the most part, conservative management should suffice. Smaller leaks may respond to stenting. If a large urinoma or infected urinoma is present, percutaneous drain or nephrostomy placement may be necessary. Failure to resolve with conservative management may require open exploration/ repair. If intraoperative suspicion of renal pelvic leak exists, methylene blue can be administered intravenously. Prevention of renal pelvic leak would be assisted by ureteral stent placement.

Laparoscopic partial nephrectomy is now becoming an established alternative for small renal tumors. With techniques duplicating open surgical principles, Gill et al. (15) found a urine leak after laparoscopic partial nephrectomy in 2% of patients. Advances in tissue sealant technology such as fibrin glues could potentially help prevent urinary leak by sealing small defects in the collecting system (16).

URETHRAL INJURIES

The urethrovesical anastomosis can leak after laparoscopic prostatectomy. In their series of 550 consecutive laparoscopic prostatectomies, Guillonneau and colleagues (17) noted 10% incidence of anastomotic leak. Rassweiler et al. (18) noted a urine leak incidence of 17.2% out of 180 laparoscopic prostatectomy patients.

Urine leak from the vesicourethral anastomosis can manifest as persistent postoperative drain output or urethrocutaneous fistula to a surgical incision. As with open radical prostatectomy, management is typically conservative. Maintaining Foley catheter and surgical drains may be necessary until drainage subsides. Guillonneau et al. (17) described one instance in which a urine leak patient underwent reoperation and laparoscopic revision of vesicourethral anastomosis on postoperative day 8. The presence of extravasated urine may increase likelihood of bladder neck contracture at the anastomotic site.

To prevent urethral leak, one must first ascertain that the Foley catheter is unobstructed and emptying well. Mild temporary catheter traction may help. Catheter traction must not be employed for an extended period of time as it may cause ischemia at the anastomosis. It is also possible that utilizing a running suture anastomosis instead of an interrupted one may decrease the incidence of postoperative urine leak.

CONCLUSION

In general, urine leak is a rare complication of laparoscopic surgery. Therefore, a high index of suspicion is necessary to rapidly identify and treat such injuries. It is important to be aware of the anatomic proximity of urinary tract structures to the planes of dissection. If the possibility of urinary tract injury exists, simple preventive measures are sufficient to avoid injury. Though radiographic and biochemical testing can greatly assist the clinician, the power of observation and physical exam must not be neglected in the evaluation.

One reason that urine leak is a rare complication has been the fact that most laparoscopic urology has been simple extirpative procedures such as adrenalectomy and nephrectomy. Advances in the technique and technology of laparoscopic urology are facilitating the performance of reconstructive and more extensive extirpative urologic procedures. Already, with the rapid adoption of laparoscopic prostatectomy worldwide, urine leak complications are becoming more common (17,18). With more complex reconstructive procedures now being described such as laparoscopic ileal ureter (19), ileocystoplasty (20), and ileal neobladder (21,22), we can expect that urine leak complications may become more common.

KEY POINTS

- Urine leak after laparoscopic urologic surgery is rare and usually is a consequence of reconstructive procedures.
- Intraoperative recognition of ureteral injury by other surgical specialties is important to reduce morbidity and repair requires laparoscopic suturing techniques.
- Delayed recognition of injuries may require open surgical correction.
- Decompression of the bladder with a catheter reduces the risk of bladder injury.
- Preoperatively identifying difficult cases and placement of ureteral catheters can help prevent injuries.

REFERENCES

1. Fahlenkamp D, Rassweiler J, Fornara P, Frede T, Loening SA. Complications of laparoscopic procedures in urology: experience of 2407 procedures at 4 German centers. J Urol 1999; 162(3):765–770.

2. Raju T, Steele R, Ahuja S. Complications of urological laparoscopy: a standardized 1 institution experience. J Urol 1996; 156(2):469–471.

3. Cadeddu J, Regan F, Kavoussi LR, Moore RG. The role of computerized tomography in the evaluation of complications after laparoscopic urological surgery. J Urol 1997; 158(4): 1349–1352.

4. Saidi MH, Sadler RK, Vancaillie TG, Akright BD, Farhart SA, White AJ. Diagnosis and management of serious urinary complications after major operative laparoscopy. Obstet Gynecol 1996; 87:272–276.

5. Sadik S, Onoglu AS, Mendilcioglu I, Sehirali S, Sipahi C, Taskin O, Wheeler JM. Urinary tract injuries during advanced gynecologic laparoscopy. J Am Assoc Gynecol Laparosc 2000; 7(4):569–572.

6. Tamussino KF, Lang PFJ, Breinl E. Ureteral complications with operative gynecologic laparoscopy. Am J Obstet Gynecol 1998; 178(5):967–970.

7. Oh BR, Kwon DD, Kwang SP, Ryu SB, Park YI, Presti JS. Late presentation of ureteral injury after laparoscopic surgery. Obstet Gynecol 2000; 95(3):337–339.

8. Larach SW, Patankar SK, Ferrara A, Williamson PR, Perozo SE, Lord AS. Complications of laparoscopic colorectal surgery: analysis and comparison of early vs. latter experience. Dis Colon Rectum 1997; 40(5):592–596.

9. Agachan F, Joo JS, Weiss EG, Wexner SD. Intraoperative laparoscopic complications: are we getting better? Dis Colon Rectum 1996; 39(10):S14–S19.

10. Larach SW, Gallagher JT. Complications of laparoscopic surgery for rectal cancer: avoidance and management. Semin Surg Oncol 2000; 18:265–268.

11. Mirhashemi R, Harlow BL, Ginsburg ES, Signorello LB, Berkowitz R, Feldman S. Predicting risk of complications with gynecologic laparoscopic surgery. Obstet Gynecol 1998; 92(3): 327–331.

12. Powsner RA, Edelstein RA, Jaffe T, Battinelli DL, Josephs LG. Diagnosis of postoperative urinary ascites using renal scintigraphy. Clin Nucl Med 1997; 22(8):523–525.

13. Champault G, Cazacu F, Taffinder N. Serious trochar accidents in laparoscopic surgery: a French survey of 103,852 operations. Surg Laparosc Endosc 1996; 6(5):367–370.

14. Jarrett TW, Chan DY, Charambura TC, Fugita O, Kavoussi LR. Laparoscopic pyeloplasty: the first 100 cases. J Urol 2002; 167(3):1253–1256.

15. Gill IS, Desai MM, Kaouk JH, Meraney AM, Murphy DP, Sung GT, Novick AC. Laparoscopic partial nephrectomy for renal tumor: duplicating open surgical techniques. J Urol 2002; 167:469–476.

16. Pruthi RS, Chun J, Richman M. The use of fibrin tissue sealant during laparoscopic partial nephrectomy. Br J Urol Int 2003; 93:813–817.

17. Guillonneau B, Rozet F, Cathelineau X, Lay F, Barret E, Doublet J, Baumert H, Vallancien G. Perioperative complications of laparoscopic radical prostatectomy: the Montsouris 3-year experience. J Urol 2002; 167(1):51–56.

18. Rassweiler J, Sentker L, Seeman O, Hatzinger M, Rumpelt HJ. Laparoscopic radical prostatectomy with the Heilbronn technique: an analysis of the first 180 cases. J Urol 2001; 166(6): 2101–2108.

19. Gill IS, Savage SJ, Senagore AJ, Sung GT. Laparoscopic ileal ureter. J Urol 2000; 163(4):1199–1202.

20. Elliott SP, Meng MV, Anwar HP, Stoller ML. Complete laparoscopic ileal cystoplasty. Urology 2002; 59(6):939–943.

21. Gaboardi G, Simonato A, Galli S, Lissiani A, Gregori A, Bozzola A. Minimally invasive laparoscopic neobladder. J Urol 2002; 168(3):1080–1083.

22. Gill IS, Kaouk JH, Meraney AM, Desai MM, Ulchaker JC, Klein EA, Savage SJ, Sung GT. Laparoscopic radical cystectomy and continent orthotopic ileal neobladder performed completely intracorporeally: the initial experience. J Urol 2002; 13–18.

10

Complications of Organ Extraction

OSCAR FUGITA

Division of Surgery,
University of São Paulo,
São Paulo, Brazil

INTRODUCTION

During the last decade, there has been a remarkable increase in the application of laparoscopic surgical techniques to treat urologic diseases. This approach offers the potential advantages of less postoperative pain, a shorter hospital stay, more rapid recovery, an improved cosmetic result, and a reduced cost of therapy (1–3). Since its first utilization, laparoscopic surgical technology has progressed in optical instruments, tissue dissection, endoscopic suturing techniques, as well as specimen extraction tools.

Complications of organ extraction in urologic laparoscopic surgery are rare but have been reported. Fahlenkamp et al. (4), in a multiinstitutional review of 2407 laparoscopic procedures in urology, reported a total of 107 complications (4.4%). Despite the fact that the complications were related to procedures with different degrees of technical difficulties, none of them was related to the organ extraction. Soulie et al. (5) reviewed the complications in 350 urologic laparoscopic procedures at a single center. A total of 19 (5.4%) complications occurred in this series. Correlation of complications with the laparoscopic procedural steps showed that none of them was related to the organ extraction. Vallancien et al. (6) reviewed 1311 laparoscopic urologic surgeries at a single center. A total of 3.6% intraoperative complications were observed, including major (0.7%), intermediate (1.9%), and minor (1%) complications. One patient presented with injury to the ileum while removing the bag containing the prostate after radical prostatectomy. The injury was sutured laparoscopically and the authors reported that the injury could be related to the fact that the patient awoke during the bag extraction and pushed strongly.

The issues related to organ extraction are hernia formation, organ injury, difficult specimen entrapment, port site tumor recurrences, tumor spillage, and tumor control. Several of these topics will be addressed in this chapter.

INTACT EXTRACTION VS. MORCELLATION

Removal of solid organs can be performed either intact (after placement inside a bag and brought out through an incision) or morcellated within a bag and the fragments extracted. Two important advances in this field are the development of special entrapment devices to remove the surgical specimen and the use of tissue morcellators for specimen removal through small incisions.

Retrieval of specimens via morcellation has some theoretical advantages over removal of intact specimens such as reduced risk of hernia formation (7), decrease in hospital stay and postoperative analgesic requirements (8), and a better cosmetic result. On the other hand, some major concerns with morcellation include longer operative time, injury to abdominal organs during morcellation, staging difficulties, potential for port site tumor recurrence, and long-term tumor control. Endoscopic devices that aid in specimen entrapment utilize materials for the bag that could be punctured during morcellation. Only a nylon reinforced entrapment sac (Lap Sac, Cook, Spencer, IN) is considered safe and morcellation of tumor specimens must be performed carefully. Safeguards to prevent complications are listed in Table 1.

In two separate prospective studies evaluating intact vs. morcellated specimen removal, operating time, postoperative recovery, and pathologic staging issues were compared. Gettman et al. (9) found that although extraction incision length (7.6 vs. 1.2 cm, $p < 0.05$) was significantly different between the groups, there were no differences in pain or activity scores, nor time to return to normal activity. The results from Hernandez et al. were similar with no difference in surgical time, pain, or hospital stay. Two of the 23 specimens extracted intact had a pathologic stage higher than the clinical stage (clinical T1 to pathologic T3a); however, no change in patient treatment was made based on this information (10).

The method of specimen extraction remains controversial and is dependent on the experience and preference of each surgeon.

COMPLICATIONS DURING LIVE DONOR NEPHRECTOMY

Laparoscopic living donor nephrectomy (LDN) is becoming the standard of care for renal procurement with decreased donor morbidity and equivalent recipient outcomes (11). The majority of live donor nephrectomies are performed using pure laparoscopy and an endoscopic bag device for kidney removal. Despite the increasing experience achieved at some centers, technical difficulties associated with the procedure still remain, particularly related to the kidney entrapment and removal. Sasaki et al. (12) described one case in a series of 100 LDNs in which the retrieved kidney fell out of the extraction bag, leading to 10 min of warm ischemia. Nakache et al. (13) described a case involving a large kidney that was

Table 1   Safeguards to Minimize Risk of Trocar Site Metastasis

A. Minimize direct handling of an organ that harbors a malignancy and maintain the widest surgical margin as possible

B. Organ retrieval is performed only with approved laparoscopic entrapment sacks

C. Organ morcellation performed only in conjunction with a nylon-reinforced entrapment sack (Lap Sac, Cook, Spencer, IN)

   1. When morcellation is planned, fill entrapment sack with saline before use to test for sack perforations
   2. Introduce the Lap Sac only with the approved metal introducers
   3. Use only atraumatic forceps to grasp the tabs located at the neck of the sack
   4. Drape the area around the entrapment bag during morcellation
   5. Morcellation is preferably performed with ring forceps
   6. Monitor morcellation laparoscopically if possible to minimize risk of injury
   7. Place upward traction on entrapment sack during morcellation
   8. Instruments used in conjunction with morcellation are passed off the surgical field when morcellation finished
   9. Entire operating room team changes gloves after morcellation step is completed
   10. Avoid morcellation for tumors $> 10 \, cm$ and in presence of ascites

D. Apply povidone-iodine to trocar sites at time of careful closure

difficult to entrap, leading to prolonged warm ischemia. Similarly, Rosin et al. (14) reported difficult specimen entrapment due to a tear in the collecting bag. Jacobs et al. (15) reported that unanticipated manual extraction was required in five cases of 320 LDNs (1.5%) because of failure to entrap the kidney in the extraction bag. Kavoussi (16) also reported that technical difficulties while retrieving the kidney using the EndoCatch (US Surgical, Norwalk, CT) bag have resulted in prolonged warm ischemia time. Shalhav et al. (17) described two complications related to the EndoCatch device in 43 LDNs: a splenic laceration that required splenectomy on postoperative day 1 and another case in which the kidney slipped out of the bag during removal. The kidney was manually retrieved with a resultant warm ischemia of 6 min. The kidney functioned well without sequelae.

Based on the technical problems experienced by some groups with extraction bags, some transplantation groups advocate the use of hand-assisted laparoscopy (18) or manual extraction after pure laparoscopic techniques (17). However, problems related to the cost of the hand-assisted devices, wound cosmesis, and incisional pain remain (19–21).

COMPLICATIONS DURING RADICAL NEPHRECTOMY

Laparoscopic radical nephrectomy (LRN) offers the advantages of minimally invasive surgery with decreased postoperative analgesia requirements, shorter length of hospital stay, and faster resumption of normal activity compared with the traditional open approach (1,2). Data on the advantages of morcellation of LRN specimens over intact specimen removal in regards to analgesic requirements and time of hospital stay are controversial (22,23). On the other hand, technical difficulties have been experienced by some groups. During a pilot study of cytoreductive LRN, placement of large tumors into a sac before morcellation took a median time of 39 min (22). The retrieval of large specimens after morcellation also carries the potential of enlarging the fascia incision. The specimen pieces must be grasped and extracted multiple times and in so doing, the fascia may be stretched and torn. Richter's hernia related to this activity has been reported (7). Also, morcellators cut through tissue by rotating a sharp blade against the specimen. Injury to adjacent structures may occur if they are brought into the morcellator's cylinder while the blade is rotating.

Other major concerns regarding morcellation after LRN are related to port site seeding, inadequate tumor control, and preservation of staging information (8,24,25). The last aspect may be considered a limitation of the morcellation technique but not a true complication.

PORT SITE SEEDING

Trocar site metastasis is a significant postoperative complication, especially in the gynecology and general surgery literature (26,27). In the urologic literature, only one patient has been reported to develop a trocar recurrence after laparoscopic pelvic lymph node dissection (LPLND) for prostate cancer (28); however, the incidence of port site recurrence following LPLND for transitional cell cancer (TCC) of the bladder is approximately 4% (29). A propensity for subcutaneous tumor recurrence has also been reported following percutaneous resection of TCC, a procedure utilizing access methods analogous to laparoscopy (30–32). The issue of port site recurrence, however, is even more concerning as laparoscopic management of renal cell carcinoma and upper-tract TCC have evolved. To date, at least three patients have developed port site recurrence following laparoscopic nephrectomy for RCC and at least two patients have developed TCC port site recurrence after laparoscopic nephroureterectomy (33–37). In the cases of renal cancer port site recurrence, a nylon reinforced specimen bag was not used.

Trocar site metastasis has been the subject of clinical and basic science research (26,27,38). A multifactorial basis of trocar site metastasis is proposed, with biological properties of the tumor, immune status of the patient, local trauma, tumor manipulation, and surgical technique implicated in trocar seeding (39–41). Previously, pneumoperitoneum was implicated in the development of trocar site metastasis (42,43); however, the significance of this factor has been refuted in recent publications (27,44). Surgical technique has been increasingly targeted as the basis of port site recurrences (39,40). For laparoscopic resection of RCC, the safety of specimen retrieval may also represent an important contributing factor. Indeed, all cases of RCC trocar site recurrence, to date, have been associated with morcellated specimen extraction (33,35).

Port site metastases are manifested by pain, palpable mass, or skin lesion overlying the trocar incision (28,29,33,35–37). Port site metastases associated with prostate cancer, TCC, and RCC have developed postoperatively at 6 months, 3–9 months, 5–25 months, respectively (28,29,33,35–37). A metastatic survey is warranted for patients with suspected trocar site recurrences. The diagnosis is confirmed by biopsy. Treatment is guided by the results of the metastatic survey and the tumor type. For example, Fentie and colleagues (35) performed wide local excision of a solitary RCC port site recurrence resulting in a tumor-free status for the patient at 35 months after resection. In contrast, port site recurrences with TCC are commonly associated with concurrent metastasis and a poor outcome even with chemotherapy (29).

Careful laparoscopic technique and adherence to oncologic principles is warranted for the prevention of trocar site recurrences (Table 1) (22,29,34,38). With the use of appropriate safeguards, the risk of port site recurrence appears minimal; however, increased scientific investigation and clinical experience are warranted to fully understand the pathogenesis of this problem.

KEY POINTS

- Complications related to organ extraction are rare.
- In prospective published studies, no significant advantage (except for extraction incision length) is found for morcellated vs. intact specimen removal.

- The live donor nephrectomy specimen can be removed either with extraction bag devices or manually.
- Morcellation of specimens must be performed carefully using approved devices and techniques.

REFERENCES

1. McDougall EM, Clayman RV, Elashry OM. Laparoscopic radical nephrectomy for renal tumor: the Washington University experience. J Urol 1996; 155:1180–1185.

2. Ono Y, Katoh N, Kinukawa T, Matsuura O, Ohshima S. Laparoscopic radical nephrectomy: the Nagoya experience. J Urol 1997; 158:719–723.

3. Wilson BG, Deans GT, Kelly J, McCrory D. Laparoscopic nephrectomy: initial experience and cost implications. Br J Urol 1995; 75:276–280.

4. Fahlenkamp D, Rassweiler J, Fornara P, Frede T, Loening SA. Complications of laparoscopic procedures in urology: experience with 2,407 procedures at 4 German centers. J Urol 1999; 162:765–770.

5. Soulie M, Seguin P, Lsaure R, Mouly P, Vazzoler N, Pontonnier F, Plante P. Urological complications of laparoscopic surgery: experience with 350 procedures at a single center. J Urol 2001; 165:1960–1963.

6. Vallancien G, Cathelineau X, Baumert H, Doublet JD, Guilloneau B. Complications of transperitoneal laparoscopic surgery in urology: review of 1,311 procedures at a single center. J Urol 2002; 168:23–26.

7. Miller CE. Methods of tissue extraction in advanced laparoscopy. Curr Opin Obstet Gynecol 2001; 13:399–405.

8. Landman J, Lento P, Hassen W, Unger P, Waterhouse R. Feasibility of pathological evaluation of morcellated kidneys after radical nephrectomy. J Urol 2000; 164:2086–2089.

9. Gettman MT, Napper C, Corwin TS, Cadeddu JA. Laparoscopic radical nephrectomy: prospective assessment of impact of intact versus fragmented specimen removal on postoperative quality of life. J Endourol 2002; 16:23–26.

10. Hernandez F, Rha KH, Pinto PA, Kim FJ, Klicos N, Chan TY, Kavoussi LR, Jarrett TW. Laparoscopic nephrectomy: assessment of morcellation versus intact specimen extraction on postoperative status. J Urol 2003; 170:412–415.

11. Chan DY, Fabrizio MD, Ratner LE, Kavoussi LR. Complications of laparoscopic live donor nephrectomy: the first 175 cases. Transplant Proc 2000; 32:778.

12. Sasaki TM, Finelli F, Bugarin E, Fowlkes D, Trollinger J, Barhyte DY, Light JA. Is the laparoscopic donor nephrectomy the new criterion standard? Arch Surg 2000; 135:943–947.

13. Nakache R, Szold A, Merhav H, Klausner JM. Kidney graft loss after laparoscopic live donor nephrectomy. Transplant Proc 2000; 32:693.

14. Rosin D, Shabtai M, Saavedra-Malinger P, Rahamimov R, Gershoni R, Ayalon A. Laparoscopic donor nephrectomy. Transplant Proc 2000; 32:681–682.

15. Jacobs SC, Cho E, Dunkin BJ, Flowers JL, Schweitzer E, Cangro C, Fink J, Farney A, Philosophe B, Jarrell B, Bartlet ST. Laparoscopic donor nephrectomy: the University of Maryland 3-year experience. J Urol 2000; 164:1494–1499.

16. Kavoussi LR. Laparoscopic donor nephrectomy. Kidney Int 2000; 57:2175–2186.

17. Shalhav AL, Siqueira TM, Gardner TA, Paterson RF, Stevens LH. Manual specimen retrieval without a pneumoperitoneum preserving device for laparoscopic live donor nephrectomy. J Urol 2002; 168:941–944.

18. Wolf JS, Tchetgen MB, Merion RM. Hand-assisted laparoscopic live donor nephrectomy. Urology 1998; 52:885–887.

19. Rudich SM, Marcovich R, Magee JC, Punch JD, Campbell DA, Merion RM, Konnak JW, Wolf JS. Hand-assisted laparoscopic donor nephrectomy: comparable donor/recipient outcomes, costs, and decreased convalescence as compared to open donor nephrectomy. Transplant Proc 2001; 33:1106–1107.

20. McGinnis DE, Gomella LG, Strup SE. Comparison and clinical evaluation of hand-assist devices for hand-assisted laparoscopy. Tech Urol 2001; 7:57–61.

21. Kim FJ, Ratner LE, Kavoussi LR. Renal transplantation: laparoscopic live donor nephrectomy. Urol Clin North Am 2000; 27:777–785.

22. Walther MM, Lyne JC, Libutti SK, Linehan WM. Laparoscopic cytoreductive nephrectomy as preparation for administration of systemic interleukin-2 in the treatment of metastatic renal cell carcinoma: a pilot study. Urology 1999; 53:496–501.

23. Dunn M, Portis A, Shalhav A, Elbahnasy AM, Heidorn C, McDougall EM, Clayman RV. Laparoscopic versus open radical nephrectomy: a 9-year experience. J Urol 2000; 164:1153–1159.

24. Rabban JT, Meng MV, Yeh B, Koppie T, Ferrell L, Stoller M. Kidney morcellation in laparoscopic nephrectomy for tumor: recommendations for specimen sampling and pathological tumor staging. Am J Surg Pathol 2001; 25:1158–1166.

25. Caddedu JA, Ono Y, Clayman RV, Barrett PH, Janetschek G, Fentie DD, McDougall EM, Moore RG, Kinukawa T, Elbahnasy AM, Nelson JB, Kavoussi LR. Laparoscopic nephrectomy for renal cell cancer: evaluation of efficacy and safety: a multicenter experience. Urology 1998; 52:773–777.

26. Paolucci V, Schaeff B, Schneider M, Gutt C. Tumor seeding following laparoscopy: international survey. World J Surg 1999; 23:989–995.

27. Tsivian A, Shtabsky A, Issakov J, Gutman M, Ami Sidi A, Szold A. The effect of pneumoperitoneum on dissemination and scar implantation of intra-abdominal cells. J Urol 2000; 164:2096–2098.

28. Bangma CH, Kirkels WJ, Chada S, Schroder FH. Cutaneous metastasis following laparoscopic pelvic lymphadenectomy for prostatic carcinoma. J Urol 1995; 153:1635–1636.

29. Elbahnasy AM, Hoenig DM, Shalhav A, McDougall EM, Clayman RV. Laparoscopic staging of bladder tumor: concerns about port site metastases. J Endourol 1998; 12:55–59.

30. Huang A, Low RK, deVere White R. Nephrostomy tract tumor seeding following percutaneous manipulation of a ureteral carcinoma. J Urol 1998; 153:1041–1042.

31. Sharma NK, Nicol A, Powell CS. Track infiltration following percutaneous resection of renal pelvic transitional cell carcinoma. Br J Urol 1994; 73:597–598.

32. Doret M, Mege JL, Fendler JP, Kepenekian G. Parietal metastasis in nephrectomy track reveals pyelic transitional cell carcinoma. J Urol 2001; 165:520.

33. Castilho LN, Fugita OEH, Mitre AI, Arap S. Port site tumor recurrences of renal cell carcinoma after videolaparoscopic radical nephrectomy. J Urol 2001; 165:519.

34. Landman J, Clayman RV. Letter. J Urol 2001; 166:629–630.

35. Fentie DD, Barrett PH, Taranger LA. Metastatic renal cell cancer after laparoscopic radical nephrectomy: long-term follow-up. J Endourol 2000; 14:407–411.

36. Ahmed I, Shaikh NA, Kapadia CR. Track recurrence of renal pelvic transitional cell carcinoma after laparoscopic nephrectomy. Br J Urol 1998; 81:319.

37. Otani M, Irie S, Tsuji Y. Port site metastasis after laparoscopic nephrectomy: unsuspected transitional cell carcinoma within a tuberculous atrophic kidney. J Urol 1999; 162:486–487.

38. Urban DA, Kerbl K, McDougall EM, Stone AM, Fadden PT, Clayman RV. Organ entrapment and renal morcellation: permeability studies. J Urol 1993; 150:1792–1794.

39. Reymond MA, Schneider C, Kastl S, Hohenberger W, Kockerling F. The pathogenesis of port-site recurrences. J Gastrointest Surg 1998; 2:406–414.

40. Schneider C, Jung A, Reymond MA, Tannapfel A, Balli J, Franklin ME, Hohenberger W, Kockerling F. Efficacy of surgical measures in preventing port-site recurrences in a porcine model. Surg Endosc 2001; 15:121–125.

41. Neuhaus SJ, Watson DI, Ellis T, Rofe AM, Jamieson GG. The effect of immune enhancement and suppression on the development of laparoscopic port site metastases. Surg Endosc 2000; 14:439–443.

42. Bouvy ND, Marquet RL, Jeekel H, Bonjer HJ. Impact of gas(less) laparoscopy and laparotomy on peritoneal tumor

growth and abdominal wall metastases. Ann Surg 1996; 224:694–700.

43. Mathew G, Watson DI, Ellis T, DeYong N, Rofe AM, Jamieson GG. The effect of laparoscopy on the movement of tumor cells and metastasis to surgical wounds. Surg Endosc 1997; 11:1163–1166.

44. Tomita H, Marcello PW, Milson JW, Gramlich TL, Fazio VW. CO2 pneumopertoneum does not enhance tumor growth and metastasis: a study of a rat cecal wall inoculation model. Dis Colon Rectum 2001; 44:1297–1301.

11

Hernia

PETER COLEGROVE and SANJAY RAMAKUMAR
University of Arizona Health Sciences Center,
Tucson, Arizona, U.S.A.

INCIDENCE

Trocar hernias are an increasingly reported, yet largely avoidable, postoperative complication of laparoscopic access (1). Poor closure of a trocar incision (or not attempting closure at all) is the main contributing factor in the development of a trocar hernia (1–3). Trocar hernias can increase the morbidity of an otherwise uncomplicated minimally invasive surgical procedure. Trocar hernias most commonly occur through fascial incisions that are $\geq 10\,mm$ in length; however, hernias have also occurred at $5\,mm$ trocar sites (3–6). The potential for abdominal herniation through trocar sites was first reported in 1968 early in the development of laparoscopic techniques (7). Although the development of improvements in trocar placement and fascial closure techniques have decreased the incidence of trocar hernias, the occurrence of such complications has not been eliminated completely.

In 1973, Bishop and Halpin (8) reported one of the first cases of herniation of omentum through an umbilical trocar site requiring surgical reduction. The first report of post-operative bowel herniation came soon after in 1974 by Schiff and Naftolin. They noted the incarceration of bowel in two patients after laparoscopic tubal ligation, which eventually required small bowel resection (9). Several similar case reports followed describing obstructive symptoms attributed to everything from strangulated omentum to Richter's hernias at trocar sites (10,11).

It was recognized early that the majority of hernias were occurring through large 11–12 mm port sites (8,10,11). Initial recommendations focused on decreasing the incidence of herniation by developing a "Z" tract or angled tract of trocar passage but did not suggest need for closure of the site. It was not until the early 1990s did laparoscopists begin to advocate primary closure of fascia at trocar sites 10 mm or larger (12).

The explosion of laparoscopic techniques developed within the OB/GYN and general surgical communities saw a concomitant increase in the number of reported trocar hernias. Larger series were reported in which the incidence of laparoscopic trocar hernias ranged from 0.2% to 4.9% (13–17). In the majority of these early reports, the trocar sites were not closed primarily. It is likely that the early incidence of trocar hernia was higher than in modern series because larger trocar sites are usually closed primarily. The current incidence of trocar herniation probably lies around 1%.

Primary closure of the fascial defects, however, did not completely prevent herniation. One early review by Montz et al.(16) noted that almost 18% of the hernias reported in their retrospective review occurred despite fascial closure. Kadar et al. noted that importance of adequate closure should not be underestimated. They report that in one case of trocar herniation the fascia had unequivocally been missed during attempted closure. In three of their five reported cases of trocar herniation, the surgeon attempted to close the fascia. These authors advocated the development of devices to facilitate the en-bloc closure of laparoscopic fascial defects. To that end, James Carter (18) developed the Carter–Thompson Needle Point Suture passer, which ensured complete fascial closure under direct laparoscopic vision. Several other suture devices have been developed in the interim (19).

The use of smaller port sites (5 mm) did not prevent the development of trocar site herniation either (17,20–22). Nezhat et al.(17) reported their incidence of trocar site herniations and found that almost half of their incisional hernias were at a 5 mm trocar site. Most authors have attributed this occurrence to excessive manipulation of the port site, which may widen or extend the fascial and peritoneal defect (17,20–22). They have advocated primary closure of any size port associated with excessive manipulation (22). Extension of a trocar site to allow passage of a tissue specimen has also been implicated as a risk factor for herniation. Nassar et al.(13) reported 12 of 16 (75%) incisional hernias associated with wound extension to facilitate removal of the specimen during laparoscopic cholecystectomy.

Several studies have described a higher incidence of trocar hernias in patients with preexisting hernias, especially periumbilical hernias (13,14,23,24). Azurin et al. reported that 90% of their trocar hernias were associated with a preexisting umbilical hernia. The incidence of preexisting umbilical hernias has been reported to be between 9% and 18% (13,14,23). These preexisting hernias may predispose herniation of bowel contents through trocar sites, especially if the preexisting hernia is not discovered and subsequently repaired at the time of surgery. Bergemann et al. report a case of omental herniation through a 3 mm umbilical trocar site. On exploration of the site, a previously unnoticed fascial defect lateral to the umbilical trocar site was noted. The omentum had tracked through the hernia sac and externalized at the skin incision (24). Thorough examination of the abdomen both in the preoperative and operative setting is warranted, given the increased risk of fascial dehiscence. Many have advocated a primary repair of the fascial defect at the time of surgery using nonabsorbable suture and mesh when necessary (14,23). Patients may not readily volunteer the presence of a fascial defect, as only 16–56% are symptomatic.

Associations between wound infection and port site herniation have also been described (12,14,25).

Massive obesity has been regarded as a relative contraindication for laparoscopic surgery in the past. Mendoza et al. conducted a multi-institutional review of laparoscopic complications in obese urologic patients noting a higher incidence of overall complications but only listed a single case of incisional hernia at a trocar site (0.8%). However, Matthews et al. reported a case of preperitoneal Richter's hernia in a morbidly obese patient undergoing a laparoscopic gastric bypass. They recommend incorporating the thick preperitoneal layer into the fascial closure to decrease the potential preperitoneal space (26).

UROLOGIC LITERATURE

The incidence of trocar herniation in the urologic literature has been favorably low. In 1995, Gill et al. (27) reported complications of laparoscopic nephrectomy in 185 patients from multiple institutions, noting two trocar hernias, both requiring surgical repair. Fahlenkamp et al. report complications in 2407 urologic laparoscopy procedures at 4 German centers over a similar 6-year period. They reported an overall complication rate of 4.4% with five hernias related to trocar sites (0.2%) (28). Cadeddu et al. report complication rates for 738 procedures performed by 13 urologists who had received at least 12 months of dedicated urologic training. They reported an overall complication rate of 11.9% with two (0.3%) trocar hernias (29).

Osama et al. reported an *incisional* hernia rate of 17% in patients undergoing laparoscopic nephrectomy with intact specimen removal through a flank incision. The authors have subsequently switched to a midline or subcostal incisional approach for removal of specimens (30). Jacobs et al. reported the University of Maryland experience with 320 laparoscopic live donor nephrectomies. In their review, there was a single case of an 11 mm trocar site herniation and five cases of *incisional* umbilical herniation through which the kidney was extracted (31). These complications underscore the importance of careful attention to primary closure of nonport site defects such as those created for removal of intact specimens no matter the location.

Hemal et al. (32) report their experience with 167 retroperitoneoscopic nephrectomies over a 5-year period noted a single port site hernia as a long-term complication.

Kumar et al. report complications from a series of 316 retroperitoneoscopic nephrectomies. They note a single incisional hernia discovered 4 months postop and was related to a subcutaneous abscess, which was treated by incision and healing by secondary intention. The authors suggest that the retroperitoneal approach may provide protection against hernia formation (33).

RECOGNITION

The most adverse consequence of a trocar hernia is the concurrent development of bowel obstruction (26). In this situation, a "ring" defect in the abdominal wall permits development of a Richter hernia (34). Nausea, bloating, and vague cramping abdominal pain frequently accompany this complication, but some patients also complain of localized trocar site discomfort (26,35). Richter hernias become manifest 2–10 days after surgery (3,26,36). Because only a portion of bowel is entrapped in the defect, classic symptoms of bowel obstruction are absent or delayed (26). Clinical findings alone often mandate exploration; however, computerized tomography or standard upper gastrointestinal contrast studies can provide important diagnostic information (37). The presence of incarcerated bowel requires immediate open or laparoscopic repair (5,26). Depending on the appearance of the bowel and the duration of obstruction, bowel resection or diverting enterostomy may be required (36). If concerns arise regarding the bowel, consultation with general surgery is recommended.

Early signs and symptoms of trocar herniation have been wide and varied. Because of relatively short postoperative stays, many patients have presented shortly after discharge (38). Boike et al. performed a multi-institutional review of incidence of bowel herniation after laparoscopic gynecologic procedures. Of the 22 cases, 18 were small bowel, two cecum, and one ascending colon. The average interval to operative intervention was 8.5 days. The diagnosis was made by CT in eight, clinical exam in six, and abdominal series in three (39). The majority of reviews described patients presenting within 10 days (38–40), although trocar hernias have reported as far out as 2 years after surgery (23). As the initial presentation can be quite varied, early clinical suspicion of a hernia can greatly improve time to diagnosis. Signs and symptoms may include complaints of abdominal pain, nausea, vomiting, diarrhea, fevers, chills, and other constitutional symptoms. Physical exam may demonstrate swelling or erythema at the incision site, abdominal distention, or present as a relatively benign abdomen.

Imaging studies obtained largely depend on index of suspicion and presenting symptoms. Differentiation between bowel obstruction and paralytic ileus in the immediate postoperative period can be difficult. Several case reports have stated that CT imaging may be helpful in diagnosing incisional hernias (37,41). Frager et al. conducted a prospective study comparing CT vs. clinical exam and plain film radiographic findings for diagnosis. They demonstrated that CT findings were 100% sensitive in definitively diagnosing small bowel obstruction in comparison to 19% sensitivity for clinical exam and plain film findings (42).

For patients with signs of a bowel obstruction where no clear fascial defect is identified, the possibility of an internal especially mesenteric hernia should be considered (Figs. 1 and 2). Small bowel obstruction due to incarcerated small bowel through the large bowel mesentery is a possibility. CT scan is helpful in making the diagnosis. The authors brought attention to the possibility of this problem as well as the need to close all mesenteric defects (even large bowel) during procedures (43).

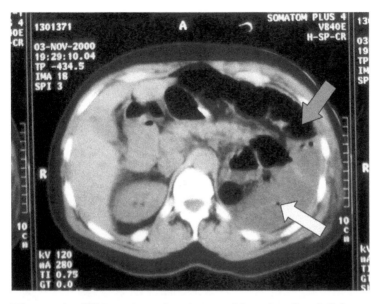

Figure 1   CT imaging of an internal hernia after left laparoscopic radical nephrectomy. Dilated small bowel (yellow arrow) is seen posterior to the descending colon (red arrow). (*See color insert*)

MANAGEMENT STRATEGIES

If patients present with symptoms of ileus in the immediate postoperative setting, bowel rest is recommended. If symptoms do not improve within 24 hr, a CT is recommended to help define the etiology of the ailment. Once an incisional hernia is diagnosed, repair can be accomplished through a formal laparotomy or with laparoscopy. If a large fascial defect is present, then a formal herniorrhaphy should be performed. Bowel resection of the affected portion may be required.

PREVENTION TECHNIQUES

Prior to the laparoscopic procedure, all preexisting fascial defects, especially at the umbilicus, should be identified. The hernia should be included in the closure of the trocar site (if small) or formally repaired. All fascial defects 10 mm or greater should be considered for closure. Radially dilating

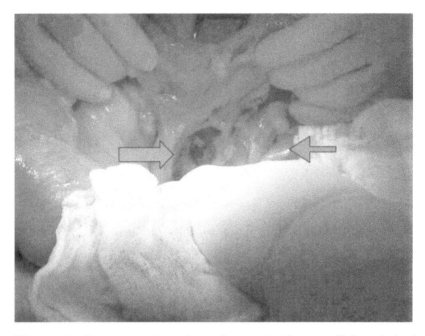

Figure 2 Intraoperative photo demonstrating small bowel (red arrow) reduced from the defect in the descending colon mesentery (green arrow). Small bowel resection was not necessary. (*See color insert*)

trocars appear to prevent trocar hernias; however, additional clinical experience with these devices is warranted (44,45). All port sites with excessive manipulation tend to have widened fascial defects and are best closed. In pediatric cases, 5 mm ports should be closed as well. Ensure that the fascia is properly closed. Devices such as the Carter–Thompson needle passer facilitate proper closure under direct visualization. Elashry et al. (19) compared eight fascial closure devices or techniques in a prospective, randomized fashion and found the Carter–Thompson port-closure technique to be their preferred method of closure. In obese patients with a large preperitoneal space created by the surgery, the fat should be reapproximated to eliminate another potential space for herniation. Examine the mesentery for any defects and close the defect with suture if identified. Finally, meticulous closure of incisional defects used to remove specimens and prevention of wound infections will decrease hernia formation.

KEY POINTS

- Poor closure of trocar sites is the leading contributor to port site hernias.
- All defects 10 mm in adults (5 mm in children) or greater should be closed.
- Mesenteric defects must be repaired to prevent internal hernia.
- Fascial closure devices facilitate proper reapproximation of tissue.

REFERENCES

1. Mayol J, Garcia-Aguilar J, Ortiz-Oshiro E, De-Diego Carmona JA, Fernandez-Represa JA. Risks of the minimal access approach for laparoscopic surgery: multivariate analysis of morbidity related to umbilical trocar insertion. World J Surg 1997; 21:529–533.

2. Hashizume M, Sugimachi K. Study Group of Endoscopic Surgery in Kyushu, Japan. Needle and trocar injury during laparoscopic surgery. Surg Endosc 1997; 11:1198–1201.

3. Eltabbakh GH. Small bowel obstruction secondary to herniation through a 5-mm laparoscopic trocar site following laparoscopic lymphadenectomy. Eur J Gynaecol Oncol 1999; 20: 275–276.

4. Plaus WJ. Laparoscopic trocar site hernia. J Laparoendosc Surg 1993; 3:567–570.

5. Romagnolo C, Minelli L. Small-bowel occlusion after operative laparoscopy: our experience and review of the literature. Endoscopy 2001; 33:88–90.

6. Nakajima K, Wasa M, Kawahara H, Hasegawa T, Soh H, Taniguchi E, Ohashi S, Okada A. Revision laparoscopy for incarcerated hernia at a 5-mm trocar site following pediatric

laparoscopic surgery. Surg Laparosc Endosc Percutan Tech 1999; 9:294–295.

7. Fear RE. Laparoscopy: a valuable aid in gynecologic diagnosis. Am J Obstet Gynecol 1968; 31:297–309.

8. Bishop HL, Halpin TF. Dehiscence following laparoscopy: report of an unusual complication. Am J Obstet Gynecol 1979; 116:585–586.

9. Schiff I, Naftolin F. Small bowel incarceration after uncomplicated laparoscopy. Obstet Gynecol 1974; 43:674–675.

10. Bourke JB. Small-intestinal obstruction from a Richter's hernia at the site of insertion of a laparoscope. BMJ 1977; 26:1393–1394.

11. Sauer M, Jarrett JC. Small bowel obstruction following diagnostic laparoscopy. Fert Steril 1984; 42:653–654.

12. Lajer H, Widecrantz S, Heisterberg L. Hernias in trocar ports following abdominal laparoscopy. Acta Obstet Gynecol Scand 1997; 76:389–393.

13. Nassar AH, Ashkar KA, Rashed AA, Abdulmoneum MG. Laparoscopic cholecystectomy and the umbilicus. Br J Surg 1997; 84:630–633.

14. Ramachandran CS. Umbilical hernial defects encountered before and after abdominal laparoscopic procedures. Int Surg 1998; 83:171–173.

15. Regardas FSP, Rodrigues LV, Nicodemo AM, Siebra JA, Furtado DC, Regadas SMM. Complications in laparoscopic colorectal resection: main types and prevention. Surg Laparosc Endosc 1998; 8:189–192.

16. Montz FJ, Holschneider CH, Munro MG. Incisional following laparoscopy: a survey of the American association of gynecologic laparoscopists. Obstet Gynecol 1994; 84:881–884.

17. Nezhat C, Nezhat F, Seideman DS, Nezhat C. Incisional hernias after operative laparoscopy. J Laparoendosc Adv Surg Tech A 1997; 7:111–115.

18. Carter JE. A new technique of fascial closure for laparoscopic incisions. J Laparoendosc Surg 1994; 4:1143–1148.

19. Elashry OM, Giusti G, Nadler RB, McDougall EM, Clayman RV. Incisional hernia after laparoscopic nephrectomy with intact specimen removal: caveat emptor. J Urol 1997; 158:363–369.

20. Kwok A, Lam A, Ford R. Incisional hernia in a 5 mm laparoscopic port site incision. Aust N Z L Obstet Gynaecol 2000; 40:104–106.

21. Reardon PR, Preciado A, Scarborough T, Matthewa B, Marti JL. Hernia at 5-mm laparoscopic port site presenting as early postoperative small bowel obstruction. J Laparoendosc Adv Surg Tech A 1999; 9:523–525.

22. Kulacoglu IH. Regarding: Small bowel obstruction and incisional hernia after laparoscopic surgery: should 5-mm trocar sites be sutured? J Laparoendosc Adv Surg Tech A 2000; 10:227–228.

23. Azurin DJ, Go LS, Arroyo LR, Kirkland ML. Trocar site herniation following laparoscopic cholecystectomy and the significance of an incidental preexisting umbilical hernia. Am Surg 1995; 8:718–720.

24. Bergemann JL, Hobbert ML, Harkins G, Narvaez J, Asato A. Omental herniation through a 3-mm umbilical trocar site: unmasking a hidden umbilical hernia. J Laparoendosc Adv Tech 2001; 11:171–173.

25. Jones DB, Soper NJ. Complications of laparoscopic cholecystectomy. Annu Rev Med 1996; 47:31–44.

26. Matthews BD, Heniford BT, Sing RF. Preperitoneal Richter hernia after a laparoscopic gastric bypass. Surg Laparosc Endosc 2001; 11:47–49.

27. Gill IS, et al. Complications of laparoscopic nephrectomy in 185 patients: a multi-institutional review. J Urol 1995; 154:479–483.

28. Fahlenkamp D, Rassweiler J, Forama P, Frede T, Loening SA. Complications of laparoscopic procedures in urology: experience with 2407 procedures at 4 German centers. J Urol 1999; 162:765–771.

29. Cadeddu JA, Wolfe JS, Nakada S, Chen R, Shalhav A, Bishoff JT, Hamilton B, Schulman PG, Dunn M, Hoenig D, Fabrizo M,

Hedican S, Averch TD. Complications of laparoscopic procedures after concentrated training in urological laparoscopy. J
Urol 2001; 166:2109–2111.

30. Elashry OM, Nakada SY, Wolf JS, Figenshau RS, McDougall
    EM, Clayman RV. Comparative clinical study of port-closure
    techniques following laparoscopic surgery. J Am Coll Surg
    1996; 183:335–344.

31. Jacobs SC. Laparoscopic live donor nephrectomy; the uni-
    versity of Maryland 3-year experience. J Urol 2000; 164:
    1494–1499.

32. Hemal AK, Gupta NP, Wadhwa SN, Goel A, Kumar R. Retro-
    peritoneoscopic npehrectomy and nephroureterectomy for
    benign nonfunctioning kidneys: a single-center experience.
    Urology 2001; 57:644–649.

33. Kumar M, Kumar R, Hemal AK, Gupta NP. Complications of
    retroperitoneoscopic surgery at one center. Br J Urol Int
    2001; 87:607–612.

34. Philips PA, Amaral JF. Abdominal access complications in
    laparoscopic surgery. J Am Coll Surg 2001; 192:525–536.

35. Soulie M, Seguin P, Richeux L, Mouly P, Vazzoler N, Ponton-
    nier F, Plante P. Urological complications of laparoscopic sur-
    gery: experience with 350 procedures at a single center. J Urol
    2001; 165:1960–1963.

36. Williams MD, Flowers SS, Fenoglio ME, Brown TR. Richter
    hernia: a rare complication of laparoscopy. Surg Laparosc
    Endosc 1995; 5:419–421.

37. Bemporad JA, Zreik TG, Brink JA. Laparoscopic hernias: two
    case reports and a review of the literature. J Comput Assist
    Tomogr 1999; 23:86–89.

38. Puls LE, Henderson RC. Small bowel herniation after laparo-
    scopic assisted vaginal hysterectomy. Acta Obstet Gynecol
    Scand 1995; 74:307–309.

39. Boike GM, Miller CE, Spirtos NM, Mercer LJ, Fowler JM,
    Summitt R, Orr JW. Incisonal bowel herniations after opera-
    tive laparoscopy: a series of nineteen cases and review of the
    literature. Am J Obstet Gynecol 1995; 172:1726–1733.

40. Kadar N, Reich H, Liue CY, Manko GF, Gimpelson R. Incisional hernias after laparoscopic gynecologic procedures. Am J Obstet Gynecol 1993; 168:1493–1496.

41. Maio A, Ruchman RB. CT diagnosis of postlaparoscopic hernia. J Comput Assist Tomogr 1991; 15:1054–1055.

42. Frager DH, Baer JW, Bossart PA. Distinction between postoperative ileus and mechanical small-bowel obstruction: value of ct compared with clinical and other radiographic findings. AJR 1995; 164:891–894.

43. Knoepp L, Smith M, Huey J, Mancino A, Barber H. Transplantation 1999; 68(3):3449–3451.

44. Schulam PG, Hedican SP, Docimo SG. Radially expanding trocar system for open laparoscopic access. Urology 1999; 54: 727–729.

45. Termanian AM. A trocarless, reusable, visual-access cannula for safer laparoscopy; an update. J Am Assoc Gynecol Laparosc 1998; 5:1434–1438.

12

Complications of Hand-Assisted Laparoscopic Renal Surgery

LI-MING SU

James Buchanan Brady Urological
Institute, Johns Hopkins Medical
Institutions, Baltimore, Maryland, U.S.A.

R. ERNEST SOSA

The New York Presbyterian
Hospital, Joan and Sanford I. Weill
Medical College, New York
New York, U.S.A.

INTRODUCTION

A decade has past since the first reports of successful laparoscopic nephrectomy by Clayman and colleagues in 1991 (1).
During this time, indications for laparoscopic surgery within
the genitourinary tract have rapidly expanded from extirpative surgeries such as pelvic lymphadenectomy, simple and
radical nephrectomy, nephroureterectomy, and donor nephrectomy to more complex reconstructive procedures such as
pyeloplasty, radical prostatectomy, and radical cystoprosta-
tectomy with diversion. As the complexity of the surgeries

has increased, so have the technical demands on the surgeon, reflected by the long operative times and steep learning curve commonly associated with these procedures. Until recently, the routine delivery of advanced laparoscopic procedures has remained part of the armamentarium of only a relatively small number of urologists who possess the necessary laparoscopic expertise and experience to successfully accomplish these challenging tasks. This has left many urologists searching for ways of acquiring the necessary skills to provide their patients with state-of-the-art, minimally invasive surgery. Hand-assisted laparoscopy (HAL) has succeeded to this end, by shortening the learning curve for inexperienced laparoscopists, as well as helping those already versed in laparoscopy to accomplish even the most challenging of surgical procedures.

The uses of a surgeon's finger placed through a trocar site reported by Winfield et al. (2), and insertion of a gloved hand reported by Tschada et al. (3) were some of the earliest examples of hand-assisted laparoscopy. By 1996, Nakada et al. (4) reported on the first successful hand-assisted laparoscopic nephrectomy in a human using the Pneumo Sleeve device (Dexterity, Blue Bell, PA). In hand-assisted laparoscopy, the surgeon maintains the use of the most efficient and versatile tool, the human hand. By placing the nondominant hand (in general) into the abdominal cavity, the surgeon is provided with tactile feedback of surrounding vital organs and is aided in maintaining a three-dimensional spatial orientation during laparoscopic dissection. Similar results obtained with conventional laparoscopy, patients have enjoyed comparable outcomes and reduced short-term morbidity (e.g., postoperative pain, length of hospital stay, convalescence) with hand-assisted techniques when compared to open surgery.

The types of complications that occur with hand-assisted laparoscopy are in general comparable to that of conventional laparoscopy. Herein, the incidence and array of complications associated with the most common hand-assisted laparoscopic renal surgeries including radical nephrectomy, partial nephrectomy, nephroureterectomy, and live donor nephrectomy will be outlined. In addition, surgeon "morbidity" during HAL will be discussed briefly.

HAL RADICAL NEPHRECTOMY

The role of hand-assisted laparoscopy in the field of urology was first established with nephrectomy. Shortly following the first report of HAL nephrectomy in 1996 (4), Wolf and colleagues (5) published a comparison between HAL and conventional laparoscopic nephrectomies, which included 15 simple and four radical nephrectomies, and two nephroureterectomies. In this study, 13 HAL nephrectomies with intact specimen extraction were compared with eight conventional laparoscopic nephrectomies with mechanical morcellation of the specimen. Mean operative time favored the HAL group (240 vs. 325 min, $p = 0.04$), with comparable results in terms of time to first oral intake, hospital stay, pain medication requirement, and postoperative pain scores when compared to those patients undergoing standard laparoscopy. Only one major complication (one of 13, 8%) occurred in the HAL group involving a repair of a symptomatic inguinal hernia contralateral to the side of the original nephrectomy. Three major complications (three of eight, 38%) occurred in the conventional laparoscopic group including open flank reexploration for a large retroperitoneal hematoma, exploratory laparotomy for an internal omental herniation, and transient rhabdomyolysis. The overall difference in the incidence of major complications between the HAL and conventional group was not statistically significant ($p = 0.10$). Only two patients in the series required transfusions, both of whom were in the conventional laparoscopic group. Despite the comparison of only a small number of patients with unequal distribution of types of procedures between the two groups, Wolf's findings suggested that HAL facilitated laparoscopic nephrectomy with significantly decreased operative time but without a significant increase in patient morbidity as compared with standard laparoscopic techniques. Their results supported the use of HAL as a tool for those urologists previously hesitant to pursue laparoscopic nephrectomy due to its technical demands.

   In a retrospective study reviewing a more comparable group of patients undergoing radical nephrectomy for suspected renal cell carcinoma, Nelson and Wolf (6) evaluated 22 HAL with 16 standard laparoscopic radical nephrectomies. Similar to the previous study by Wolf et al. (5), HAL was associated with a shorter mean operative time (205 vs. 207 min, $p = 0.0004$) and comparable hospital stay, time to first oral intake, pain scores, and quality of life scores as compared to the standard laparoscopic group. In terms of complications, 45% of HAL nephrectomies had one or more minor complications as compared to 25% of standard laparoscopic nephrectomy cases ($p = 0.31$). The incidence of having one or more major complications was 23% in the HAL group vs. 13% in the standard group ($p = 0.67$). Although not statistically significant, the authors attributed the higher number of complications in the HAL group to the relatively sicker population of HAL patients including comorbidities such as end-stage renal disease, previous liver and kidney transplantation, multiple sclerosis, as well as the HAL group having higher ASA scores, body mass index scores, and a larger mean tumor size (6.3 vs. 4.1 cm, $p = 0.006$) as compared with the standard laparoscopic group.

Interestingly, there were two cases of wound infection and one case of ventral hernia in the HAL group and none in the standard group. Although the authors did recognize the higher number of wound complications in the HAL group, no explanation was given. This difference may be attributed to the incision-related morbidity that accompanies the relatively larger incision (i.e., 6–7 cm) typically required for HAL with subsequent intact specimen extraction, as opposed to the standard laparoscopic procedure where the specimen was morcellated trough a small, preexisting trocar site (i.e., 1–1.5 cm). Reports from the general surgery literature appear to lend support to the theory that certain wound complications that occur following laparoscopy are a function of the size of the incision. In two separate comparisons between standard laparoscopic surgery and HAL for splenectomy (7) and for various colorectal diseases (8), there was no significant difference in the incidence of wound infections, incisional hernias, or postoperative ileus between the two groups. In both of these series, specimens retrieved following pure laparoscopic dissection were removed by an open incision made at the end of the dissection and not by mechanical morcellation like in the nephrectomy series reported by Nelson and Wolf (6). Therefore, it is not surprising that the incision-related morbidity is similar between the HAL and conventional laparoscopic groups in these two series since open incisions were made in both groups to facilitate intact specimen extraction. Nevertheless, while the debate over morcellation vs. intact specimen extraction continues to fuel in the field of laparoscopic radical nephrectomy for renal cell carcinoma, only a large prospective, randomized comparison between HAL vs. pure laparoscopic dissection with mechanical morcellation of the specimen will resolve the question as to whether there is an increased incidence of wound complications following HAL radical nephrectomy.

Comparisons have also been made between HAL and open radical nephrectomy series. Nakada et al. (9) compared an equal number of HAL radical nephrectomies with a contemporary group of open radical nephrectomies. Although the mean operative time favored that of open surgery, hospital stay and convalescence were significantly shorter in the HAL group. Total complications were similar between the HAL group (three of 18, 16.7%) and open group (four of 18, 22.2%). In a similar study by Mancini et al. (10), the total complication rate was found to be 16.7% (two of 12) in each group. In both studies, there were no unique complications attributed to the use of the hand-assistance device.

HAL NEPHROURETERECTOMY

Various techniques of HAL nephroureterectomy have been described, pertaining to the management of the distal ureter and bladder cuff. Seifman et al. (11) described management of the distal ureter by one of three approaches: (1) extravesical laparoscopic dissection of the distal ureter with endoscopic stapling across the bladder cuff, (2) transurethral resection of the entire intramural ureter followed by laparoscopic nephrectomy, or (3) formal open dissection and excision of the distal ureter and bladder cuff following completion of the laparoscopic nephrectomy. Stifelman et al. (12) advocated transurethral dissection of the intramural ureter using a Collins knife. In this technique, a 5-mm laparoscopic trocar is placed through the bladder to allow for use of a laparoscopic grasper to manipulate the ureter and facilitate transurethral circumferential dissection of the intramural ureter. This was followed by HAL nephrectomy and release of the distal ureter and bladder cuff from any last remaining adventitial attachments to the bladder. Lastly, Landman and colleagues (13) used an endoscopic stapler to transect the distal ureter at the ureterovesical junction followed by transurethral unroofing and complete cauterization of the ipsilateral ureteral orifice to the level of the staples. Despite these various techniques of managing the distal ureter during HAL nephroureterectomy, there have been no reports of complications related to these procedures and specifically no recurrences in the retroperitoneum or resection site occurred at the time that these three series were published.

Similar to data published for HAL nephrectomy, comparisons have been made between HAL nephroureterectomy and open series, as well as recent comparisons with conventional laparoscopic nephroureterectomy. Seifman et al. (11) performed a prospective, nonrandomized comparison between 16 HAL and 11 open nephroureterectomies. Despite the longer operative times with HAL cases, these patients enjoyed a shorter hospital stay and a more rapid convalescence. Minor (19% vs. 45%, $p > 0.1$) and major (19% vs. 27%, $p > 0.1$) complications were comparable between the HAL and open groups. The major complications included two patients who required reintubation due to chronic obstructive pulmonary disease and one death due to cardiac arrhythmia on postoperative day 27 in the HAL group and adrenal insufficiency, cerebral vascular accident, and a febrile urinary tract infection in the open cohort. There were no unique minor or major complications attributed to the hand-assisted technique in the HAL group. In a retrospective review of 11 HAL and 11 open nephroureterectomies, Stifelman et al. (12) also reported favorable outcomes for HAL patients including reduced blood loss and shorter hospital stays as compared with the open group. Only one complication was reported in the series, which involved a prolonged ileus in one patient in the open surgery group.

Further credibility of the HAL nephroureterectomy technique is given by Landman and colleagues (13) who compared 16 HAL vs. 11 nephroureterectomies performed by standard laparoscopic techniques. Hand-assisted laparoscopy was associated with a significantly shorter operative time, with no significant difference in terms of length of hospital stay, time to oral intake, or postoperative pain when compared to conventional laparoscopic techniques. There was one open conversion in the HAL group due to failure to progress. One death also occurred in the HAL group 3 weeks after surgery in a patient who suffered cardiovascular complications, pneumonia, and reintubation following surgery due to significant comorbidities. Four postoperative complications occurred in both the HAL and conventional laparoscopic group (25% vs. 36%, respectively). Three of the four postoperative complications in the HAL group involved prolonged ileus as compared to none in the standard laparoscopic group. Although the authors offered no explanation for this observation, the increased incidence of postoperative ileus may be a consequence of increased manipulation of the bowels during the hand-assisted technique as compared to conventional laparoscopic dissection. In both the HAL and standard groups, intact specimen extraction was generally used. There were no reports of wound hernias or infections in either group.

HAL PARTIAL NEPHRECTOMY

As the number of incidental renal masses increases, so have the alternative methods used to treat these small lesions. By 1998, laparoscopic partial nephrectomy had been attempted on a total of 26 cases at various institutions (14–20). Of these 26 cases, five (19%) were converted to an open operation primarily due to inability to control hemorrhage using conventional laparoscopic means. In 2000, Wolf and colleagues (21) investigated the use of hand assistance to facilitate hemostasis during laparoscopic partial nephrectomy. They retrospectively compared 11 open partial nephrectomies with 10 laparoscopic cases, eight of which were performed using hand assistance. Selection criteria for the laparoscopic group included small (< 4 cm) and mostly peripherally located tumors. Mean lesion size was comparable between the laparoscopic and open groups (2.4 cm in both groups). Of the 10 laparoscopic cases, eight were performed using HAL (six wedge resections, two polar nephrectomies) and in two cases tumor enucleation was performed using conventional laparoscopic techniques. Hemostasis was achieved during HAL procedures with manual pressure applied onto the renal defect using a gelatin sponge soaked with fibrin glue. Vascular clamping was not used during any of the laparoscopic procedures. In the open cohort, all renal lesions were explored through an extraperitoneal flank approach with routine vascular clamping and renal cooling with ice slush. Although the mean blood loss (460 vs. 209 mL) and operative time (199 vs. 161 min) favored the open partial nephrectomy group, the differences were not statistically significant. Furthermore, there was no significant difference in the need for transfusions between the groups. All 10 laparoscopic partial nephrectomies were completed successfully without the need for open conversion. In the laparoscopic group, there were no major complications. Minor complications included postoperative urinary retention in two patients. There was one major complication in the open series involving an arteriovenous fistula that required embolization. There were no urinary leaks detected in either group. Mean length of hospitalization and return to normal activity were statistically shorter in the laparoscopic group as compared to the open group. From this study, Wolf advocated the use of HAL as a safe and minimally invasive technique of laparoscopic partial nephrectomy for all but the most exophytic renal masses, which can be managed by pure laparoscopic means.

Stifelman et al. (22) reported their technique of HAL partial nephrectomies in 11 patients. Following resection of the renal lesion, hemostatic gauze was placed over the renal defect and manual compression applied. Following this, interrupted chromic sutures were placed through the renal capsule on either side of the renal defect and across the hemostatic gauze. Lastly, Gerota's fascia was reapproximated over additional hemostatic gauze. The average blood loss was 319 mL and operative time was 273 min. One patient was converted to open surgery to ensure a negative margin in a deeply invading tumor. There were no open conversions reported due to bleeding. In this series, there were no major complications and two minor complications including an umbilical hernia and a persistent ileus requiring readmission to the hospital for intravenous hydration.

The results from these two studies would support the use of hand assistance during laparoscopic partial nephrectomy as a method of attaining prompt and effective hemostasis with manual compression without the need for clamping the renal vessels. Complications rates are low and do not appear to be technique-specific.

HAL LIVE DONOR NEPHRECTOMY

Laparoscopic live donor nephrectomy was first described in 1995 (23) and has since made great strides in reducing the morbidity of the donor patient while providing a healthy and reliable allograft for the recipient. Despite its popularity with surgeons and patients, the steep learning curve as well as the potential risks to both donor and recipient patients has limited its widespread acceptance by transplant centers around the country until recently. Hand-assisted laparoscopy has provided surgeons with a means of performing laparoscopic live donor nephrectomy with minimal donor morbidity and excellent recipient outcomes, comparable to that of both open and conventional laparoscopic series (24–26).

In 2000, Wolf and colleagues (24) reported a prospective, case-matched comparison of 10 HAL and 40 open donor nephrectomy procedures. Of note, this comparison was made using their first 10 HAL donor nephrectomy cases and thus represented their early experience with this technique. Although the operative time was longer in the HAL group, patients in this group experienced shorter hospital stays, less postoperative pain, and a shorter convalescence than that of the open cohort. More importantly, there was no significant difference in allograft function between the two groups as well as the incidence of donor complications (minor complications: HAL 30% vs. open 35%), acute rejection, delayed graft function, or ureteral complications. No major complications or transfusions were noted in the laparoscopic group as compared to the open cohort where there was one major complication involving a readmission for pyelonephritis and two patients who required blood transfusions. Even early in their experience with HAL donor nephrectomy, the authors noted no significant increase in donor morbidity with excellent recipient allograft function, comparable to that achieved with open surgery. They concluded that HAL reduces the learning curve of laparoscopic live donor nephrectomy as witnessed by the significant improvement in the mean operative time between their first and second five cases (254 vs. 177 min, $p < 0.01$).

In a larger series, Stifelman et al. (25) compared 60 HAL and 31 open live donor nephrectomies. Similar to the study by Wolf and colleagues (24), estimated blood loss, postoperative pain, length of hospital stay, and convalescence favored the HAL group. Short- and long-term recipient allograft function was comparable between the two groups. There were three (5%) major complications in the HAL group including two reexplorations, one for bleeding from a renal artery stump and another for a small bowel obstruction. The third major complication was a readmission for a persistent ileus. In the open group, there were two (6%) major complications including a pneumothorax requiring a chest tube placement and gross hematuria from a bleeding ureteral stump. In this series, the incidence of ureteral complications (one case, 2%) and delayed allograft function (one case, 2%) in the HAL group was low as compared to conventional laparoscopic series reported in the literature at the time (ureteral complications: 4.5–9%, delayed allograft function: 6.4–7.6%) (27,28).

A retrospective comparison of outcomes between open (14 cases), conventional laparoscopic (11 cases), and HAL (23 cases) live donor nephrectomy was reported in 2001 by Ruiz-Deya and colleagues (26). There were no major complications reported in the open group, two (18.2%) with conventional laparoscopy (incisional hernia, deep vein thrombosis), and three (13%) in the HAL group (two cases of ileus, open conversion for adrenal vein bleed). Unlike laparoscopic radical nephrectomy where the specimen may be morcellated, a renal allograft must be extracted intact through an open incision; therefore, one would expect the incisional morbidity to be no higher in the HAL compared to the conventional laparoscopic group. In fact, no wound infections were reported and only one case of incisional hernia occurred in the conventional laparoscopic group. Although time to oral intake was not documented in this study, the authors did suggest a slower return of bowel function due to increased bowel handling in the HAL group as evidenced by the two cases of postoperative ileus. Mean length of hospital stay, however, was not significantly longer in the HAL vs. the conventional laparoscopic group (2.0 vs. 1.6 days, $p = 0.6$). In their comparison, mean operative time (2.7 vs. 3.6 hr, $p < 0.5$) and mean warm ischemic time (1.6 vs. 3.9 min, $p < 0.5$) was significantly shorter in the HAL group as compared to the conventional laparoscopic group. Short- and long-term recipient allograft function was comparable between all three groups as was the incidence of acute rejection (open 14%, laparoscopic 9%, HAL 17%).

In conclusion, the use of HAL during live donor nephrectomy appears to provide a shorter learning curve, operative time, and warm ischemic time as compared to conventional laparoscopic techniques, with equivalent recipient outcomes. Major donor complications and recipient morbidity (including ureteral complications, acute rejection, and delayed allograft function) remain low with HAL and are comparable to that of both open and conventional laparoscopic techniques.

SURGEON "MORBIDITY" ASSOCIATED
WITH HAL

In addition to patient morbidity associated with HAL, potential technical and surgeon "morbidity" related to the use of hand-assistance devices merits mention. One of the major principles of laparoscopic surgery is the establishment and maintenance of pneumoperitoneum to provide the necessary visualization and working space for laparoscopic dissection. Loss of pneumoperitoneum may result in wasted operative time, surgeon frustration, failure to progress, open conversion, and increased morbidity. During HAL, the surgeon in general places the nondominant hand into the abdomen through an access device that maintains the necessary pneumoperitoneum by establishing a seal between the device and the surgeon's forearm. Leakage of carbon dioxide gas during HAL with first-generation devices has been somewhat problematic. During HAL nephrectomy, one group commented that gas leakage was "routine," although never enough to limit the successful completion of the operation (9). In the general surgery literature, leakage rates during HAL for various operations including colorectal surgery, splenectomy, and gastric surgery have been as high as 25–48% (8,29,30). In one series, gas leakage was significant enough to necessitate open conversion in 14% of cases (30). In a head-to-head comparison of first-generation hand-assist devices in a pig study, Stifelman and Nieder (31) concluded that none of the three commercially available devices (HandPort, Smith and Nephew, Andover, MA; Intromit, Applied Medical, Rancho Santa Margarita, CA; Pneumo Sleeve, Dexterity, Atlanta, GA) was superior to the other. No device scored greater than a 7.7 in overall satisfaction on a scale of 1–10, indicating that further modifications and refinements were needed. In the study, device failure was defined as the loss of pneumoperitoneum secondary to any components of the device, or the need to resecure the device to the abdominal wall in order to maintain pneumoperitoneum. Since then, new devices such as the LapDisc (Ethicon, Somerville, NJ) and the Gelport (Applied Medical, Rancho Santa Margarita,

CA) have been introduced and are currently awaiting critical testing.

Fatigue of the surgeon's intraperitoneal hand represents the most significant surgeon "morbidity" related to HAL surgery and can range from mild discomfort to severe cramping requiring removal of the hand to allow for resting. In a study of 68 HAL general surgery cases, Litwin et al. (29) found that hand fatigue occurred during some part of the operation in 14 (20.6%) procedures. The cause for hand fatigue can be due to many factors including incision size, length of operation, and selection of incision site for placement of the hand-assist device. The size of the incision made for the hand-assist device should on average be the surgeon's glove size in centimeters. If the incision size is made too small, this will lead to excessive compression of the surgeon's forearm by the skin and abdominal wall fascia leading to ischemia, cramping, fatigue, and pain. Hand fatigue and discomfort become even more prominent the longer the operative time. Proper placement of the incision for the hand-assist device entails selecting a site that optimizes the surgeon's ability to facilitate laparoscopic dissection of the target organ with the hand, while minimizing surgeon discomfort. The incision should be made some distance away from the target organ to allow for forward access during dissection of the organ. Placement of the incision too close to the target may impede visualization and result in awkward positioning of the surgeon's hand and inefficient dissection. The site of the incision should be made to allow for the surgeon's hand to rest in a near neutral position, thus reducing the likelihood of hand fatigue.

CONCLUSIONS

Hand-assisted laparoscopic renal surgery is associated with an acceptable occurrence of minor and major complications. In a recent multiinstitutional review of 196 HAL renal surgeries from three major academic institutions, Hedican et al. (32) reported that a total of 28 patients (14.3%) suffered 31 minor complications and 18 patients (9.2%) suffered 32

Table 1 Complications of Hand-Assisted Laparoscopic Renal Surgery

Minor complications
  Urinary retention (11)
  Minor splenic capsular injury (4)
  Ileus (4)
  Wound cellulitis (3)
  Pulmonary edema (2)
  Small bowel serosal injury (1)
  Facial/throat edema (1)
  Transient urine leak (1)
  Flank numbness (1)
  Subcutaneous abscess (1)
  Prostate bleeding (1)
  Delayed trocar hernia (1)
Major complications
  Small bowel injury (3)
  Conversion for bleeding (3), splenic injury (1), renal artery (1),
  retroperitoneal (1)
  Reintubation (3)
  Wound dehiscence (2)
  Pulmonary embolus (2)
  Prolonged intubation (2)
  Arrhythmia (2)
  Pneumonia (2)
  Internal mesenteric hernia, bowel obstruction, delayed exploration (1)
  Small bowel obstruction, delayed exploration (1)
  Major splenic injury (1)
  Myocardial infarct (1)
  Pulmonary edema (1)
  Metabolic encephalopathy (1)
  Acute renal failure requiring dialysis (1)
  Deep venous thrombosis (1)
  Retroperitoneal bleeding after heparin (1)
  Abscess (1)
  Prolonged urinary leak/stent (1)
  Fungal sepsis (1)
  Ileus (1)

Source: From Ref. 32.

major complications. The various types and incidence of minor and major complications in their study are listed in Table 1. In this preliminary report, there was no significant correlation between the incidence of complications and either patient ASA score, body mass index, surgeon's experience, or side of operation. A direct correlation was found between the patients with a history of prior abdominal or flank surgery and the incidence of intraoperative complications. Interestingly, there was a significant correlation between type of operation and incidence of intraoperative complications (nephroureterectomy: 18.9%, simple nephrectomy: 8%, live donor nephrectomy: 4%, radical nephrectomy: 1.8%, partial nephrectomy: 0%).

Wound complications such as hernias and wound infections and prolonged ileus as a result of increased manipulation of the bowels have been raised as a concern with hand-assisted laparoscopic procedures as compared to conventional techniques; however, the current series of reports suggest that the incidence of these complications is low. Larger comparative studies between conventional laparoscopy and HAL will be necessary to establish or refute these concerns.

Hand-assisted laparoscopy has provided significant inroads for urologists interested in providing their patients with minimally invasive renal surgery. Hand-assisted laparoscopy has decreased the learning curve for inexperienced laparoscopists and has even helped experienced laparoscopists accomplish complex procedures that would otherwise not be feasible by conventional laparoscopic means alone. Taken together, HAL as a technique has broadened the scope and armamentarium of laparoscopic surgery and has increased the overall surgeon pool available to deliver minimally invasive renal surgery. Patient morbidity with HAL is acceptable and at the time of this writing none of the complications appear to be related specifically to the hand-assist technique.

KEY POINTS

- The overall incidence of complications with HAL renal surgery appears comparable to that of conventional laparoscopic procedures.

- The types of complications that occur with HAL do not appear to be unique to the hand-assisted technique; however, incision-related complications (e.g., wound infection, incisional hernias) and postoperative ileus may be slightly higher following HAL procedures as compared to conventional laparoscopy.
- The morbidity associated with all types of HAL renal surgeries (i.e., radical nephrectomy, nephroureterectomy, donor nephrectomy, and partial nephrectomy) is acceptable and remains low.
- Proper planning of incision size and site can help reduce surgeon "morbidity" from hand fatigue.

REFERENCES

1. Clayman RV, Kavoussi LR, Soper NJ, Dierks SM, Merety KS, Darcy MD, Long SR, Roemer FD, Pingleton ED, Thomson PG. Laparoscopic nephrectomy: initial case report. J Urol 1991; 146:278–282.

2. Winfield HN, Chen RN, Donovan JF. Laparoscopic tricks of the trade: how to overcome lack of tactile feedback [abstr 513]. J Endourol 1996; 10:S189.

3. Tschada RK, Rassweiler JJ, Schmeller N, et al. Laparoscopic tumor nephrectomy—the German experiences. J Urol 1995; 153(suppl):479A.

4. Nakada SY, Moon TD, Gist M, Mahvi D. Use of the pneumo sleeve as an adjunct in laparoscopic nephrectomy. Urology 1996; 49:612–613.

5. Wolf JS Jr, Moon TD, Nakada SY. Hand assisted laparoscopic nephrectomy: comparison to standard laparoscopic nephrectomy. J Urol 1998; 160:22–27.

6. Nelson CP, Wolf JS Jr. Comparison of hand assisted versus standard laparoscopic radical nephrectomy for suspected renal cell carcinoma. J Urol 2002; 167:1989–1994.

7. Targarona EM, Balague C, Cerdan G, Espert JJ, Lacy AM, Visa J, Trias M. Hand-assisted laparoscopic splenectomy (HALS) in cases of splenomegaly: a comparison analysis with

conventional laparoscopic splenectomy. Surg Endosc 2002; 16:426–430.

8. HALS Study Group. Hand-assisted laparoscopic surgery vs. standard laparoscopic surgery for colorectal disease: a prospective randomized trial. Surg Endosc 2000; 14(10):896–901.

9. Nakada SY, Fadden P, Jarrard DF, Moon TD. Hand-assisted laparoscopic radical nephrectomy: comparison to open radical nephrectomy. Urology 2001; 58:517–520.

10. Mancini GJ, McQuay LA, Klein FA, Mancini ML. Hand-assisted laparoscopic radical nephrectomy: comparison with transabdominal radical nephrectomy. Am Surg 2002; 68: 151–153.

11. Seifman BD, Montie JE, Wolf JS Jr. Prospective comparison between hand-assisted laparoscopic and open surgical nephroureterectomy for urothelial cell carcinoma. Urology 2001; 57:133–137.

12. Stifelman MD, Hyman MJ, Shichman S, Sosa RE. Hand-assisted laparoscopic nephroureterectomy versus open nephroureterectomy for the treatment of transitional-cell carcinoma of the upper urinary tract. J Endourol 2001; 15:391–395.

13. Landman J, Lev RY, Bhayani S, Alberts G, Rehman J, Pattaras JG, Figenshau RS, Kibel AS, Clayman RV, McDougall E. Comparison of hand assisted and standard laparoscopic radical nephroureterectomy for the management of localized transitional cell carcinoma. J Urol 2002; 167:2387–2391.

14. Janetschek G, Daffmner P, Peschel P, Bartsch G. Laparoscopic nephron sparing surgery for small renal cell carcinoma. J Urol 1998; 159:1152–1155.

15. Gasman D, Saint F, Barthelemy Y, Antiphon P, Chopin D, Abbou CC. Retroperitoneoscopy: a laparoscopic approach for adrenal and renal surgery. Urol 1996; 47:801–806.

16. Gill IS, Delworth MG, Munch LC. Laparoscopic retroperitoneal partial nephrectomy. J Urol 1994; 152:1539–1542.

17. Luciani RC, Greiner M, Clement JC, Houot A, Didierlaurent JF. Laparoscopic enucleation of a renal cell carcinoma. Surg Endosc 1994; 8:1329–1331.

18. Winfield HN, Donovan JF, Lund GO, Kreder KJ, Stanley KE, Brown BP, Loening SA, Clayman RV. Laparoscopic partial nephrectomy: initial experience and comparison to the open surgical approach. J Urol 1995; 153:1409–1414.

19. Kageyama S, Suzuki K, Un-No T, Ushiyama T, Fujita K. Gasless laparoscopy-assisted partial nephrectomy for a complicated cystic lesion: a case report. J Endourol 1997; 11:41–44.

20. McDougall EM, Elbahnasy AM, Clayman RV. Laparoscopic wedge resection and partial nephrectomy: the Washington University experience and review of the literature. J Soc Laparoendosc Surg 1998; 2:15–23.

21. Wolf JS Jr, Seifman BD, Montie JE. Nephron sparing surgery for suspected malignancy: open surgery compared to laparoscopy with selective use of hand assistance. J Urol 2000; 163:1659–1664.

22. Stifelman MD, Sosa RE, Nakada SY, Shichman SJ. Hand-assisted laparoscopic partial nephrectomy. J Endourol 2001; 15:161–164.

23. Ratner LE, Ciseck LJ, Moore RG, Cigarroa FG, Kaufman HS, Kavoussi LR. Laparoscopic live donor nephrectomy. Transplant 1995; 60:1047–1049.

24. Wolf JS Jr, Marcovich R, Merion RM, Konnak JW. Prospective, case matched comparison of hand assisted laparoscopic and open surgical live donor nephrectomy. J Urol 2000; 163:1650–1653.

25. Stifelman MD, Hull D, Sosa RE, Su LM, Hyman M, Stubenbord W, Shichman S. Hand assisted laparoscopic donor nephrectomy: a comparison with the open approach. J Urol 2001; 166:444–448.

26. Ruiz-Deya G, Cheng S, Palmer E, Thomas R, Slakey D. Open donor, laparoscopic donor and hand assisted laparoscopic donor nephrectomy: a comparison of outcomes. J Urol 2001; 166:1270–1273.

27. Kavoussi LR. Laparoscopic donor nephrectomy. Kidney Int 2000; 57:2175–2186.

28. Ratner LE, Montgomery RA, Kavoussi LR. Laparoscopic live donor nephrectomy: the four year Johns Hopkins University experience. Nephrol Dial Transplant 1999; 14:2090–2093.

29. Litwin, DE, Darzi A, Jakimowicz J, Kelly JJ, Arvidson D, Hansen P, Callery MP, Denis R, Fowler DL, Medich DS, O'Reilly MJ, Atlas H, Himpens JM, Swanstrom LL, Arous EJ, Pattyn P, Yood SM, Ricciardi R, Sandor A, Meyers WC. Hand-assisted laparoscopic surgery (HALS) with the Hand-Port system: initial experience with 68 patients. Ann Surg 2000; 231:715–723.

30. Meyers WC. Handoscopic surgery: a prospective multicenter trial of a minimally invasive technique for complex abdominal surgery. Arch Surg 1999; 134:477–486.

31. Stifelman M, Nieder AM. Prospective comparison of hand-assisted laparoscopic devices. Urology 2002; 59:668–672.

32. Hedican SP, Wolf JS, Moon TD, Rayhill SC, Seifman BD, Nakada SY. Complications of hand-assisted laparoscopy in urologic surgery. J Urol 2002; 167(suppl):22–23.

13

Delayed Complications

OZGUR YAYCIOGLU

Department of Urology,
Baskent University School of Medicine,
Adana Clinic & Research Center,
Adana, Turkey

INTRODUCTION

It has been shown throughout the last decade that urologic laparoscopy can duplicate the efficacy of an open surgical procedure while causing lower morbidity, less postoperative pain, and shorter convalescence with improved cosmesis. Although, urologic laparoscopy is minimally invasive, it is still a major surgical procedure. The risk of complications in urologic laparoscopy can only be minimized by adhering to the basic principles that are well established and are outlined elsewhere in this book. Unfortunately, complications may occur even with the most meticulous technique. Because of the nature of laparoscopy, some complications are unrecognized during surgery and manifest in the postoperative period. These delayed complications may be hard to diagnose because of atypical symptoms. It is the aim of this chapter to review the data in the literature in order to provide thorough information and understanding of the delayed complications of urologic laparoscopic surgery and define diagnosis and management strategies.

INDICATIONS FOR REPEATED EXPLORATION

Literature Review

The incidence of complications after urologic laparoscopy are related to the difficulty of the procedure and the surgeon's experience. The complication rates are higher for more complex procedures and decrease with increasing experience of the surgeon. A multiinstitutional analysis of 2407 urologic laparoscopic procedures revealed a 0.8% overall reintervention rate (1). When the procedures are categorized, the reintervention rates were 0.0% for easy (diagnosis and therapy for cryptorchidism, varicocelectomy), 1.1% for difficult (renal cyst resection, lymphocele fenestration, pelvic lymph node dissection, nephropexy, ureteral procedures), and 2.7% for very difficult (nephrectomy, adrenalectomy, retroperitoneal lymph node dissection) procedures. Rassweiler and coworkers analyzed the relationship between the experience of the surgeon and the complication, conversion, and reintervention rates for laparoscopic nephrectomy from seven centers where more than 30 cases each were performed. The rates were 15%, 17%,and 7%, respectively, in the first 20 cases of each surgeon (140 nephrectomies) compared to 3%, 7%, and 1.7%, respectively, for the following 232 cases (2).

 Delayed complications like hematoma or lymphocele formation, urinary infection, small urinary leakage, and temporary ileus can usually be treated by conservative measures or endourologic and radiologic interventions like catheter or percutaneous drainage. Soulie and coworkers (3) analyzed the complications of urologic laparoscopic procedures in their multiinstitutional study. They reviewed data from 1085 procedures and classified complications in the groups as intraoperative, postoperative, and medical. Postoperative complications represented 52% of all complications. The most common postoperative complications were hematoma, urinoma, and wound infection at the trocar site. Hematomas occurred in 10 patients all of which were treated conservatively except for one lumbar hematoma, which was treated by percutaneous drainage at 3 months. Eight patients had retroperitoneal urinomas. All cases except one were treated with ureteral or percutaneous catheter drainage. Wound infection at the trocar site occurred in eight patients and all resolved with antibiotics. Transient paralytic ileus occurred after four laparoscopic radical prostatectomies and all resolved with nasogastric drainage and parenteral fluids. Two symptomatic lymphoceles were treated with percutaneous drainage at 2 and 3 weeks after pelvic lymphadenectomy.

Other delayed complications may ultimately necessitate repeated exploration and surgical repair. These can be classified as bowel-related, urinary, and vascular complications. Also solid organ injuries and abscess formation may necessitate management by repeated surgery. Overall rates for complications that were treated by repeated exploration have been reported as 0.7–2.8% in series that include a wide variety of urologic laparoscopic procedures (3–5). The repeated exploration rates for laparoscopic nephrectomy and laparoscopic pelvic lymph node dissection are 1.8–3.1%, and 0.7–7%, respectively (2,6–10). Table 1 shows the repeated exploration rates for delayed complications after urologic laparoscopic surgery. Overall, the repeated exploration rate is 61 in 4003 procedures (1.5%).

The most frequent complications treated by repeated surgery are bowel-related complications. Twenty-four of 61 (39.3%) repeated explorations were performed because of bowel-related complications. Eight of these cases resulted from herniation of bowel through a trocar site. Yaycioglu and coworkers (5) reported six patients who underwent repeated exploration because of bowel injury or bowel-related complications after urologic laparoscopic surgery.

Table 1 Meta-analysis of nine series in the literature for delayed complications that were managed by repeated exploration and surgical repair after urologic laparoscopic surgery

Series	Procedure	Patients	Repeated surgery (%)	Bowel injury	Urine leak	Vascular injury	Other
Yaycioglu et al. (5)	Various	1,226	9 (0.7%)	6[a]	2	2[a]	—
Soulie et al. (3)	Various	1,085	11 (1%)	3	6	2	—
Parra et al. (4)	Various	221	6 (2.8%)	2	1	—	3
Rassweiler et al. (2)	Nephrectomy	482	15 (3.1%)	3	—	7	5
Gill et al.	Nephrectomy	185	4 (2.2%)	2	—	1	2
Eraky et al. (7)	Nephrectomy	106	2 (1.8%)	1	—	1	—
Kavoussi et al. (8)	PLND	372	6 (1.6%)	3	2	—	1
Thomas et al. (9)	PLND	241	2 (0.7%)	—	1	—	1
Chow et al. (10)	PLND	85	6 (7%)	4	2	—	—
Total		4,003	61 (1.5%)	24[a]	14	12[a]	12

[a]One patient had both bowel and vascular injury.

Two patients underwent repeated laparoscopic exploration because of postoperative ileus after pyeloplasty with pyelolithotomy and ureteral reimplantation with Boari flap. In both cases, the diagnostic laparoscopy was negative. One of these patients had Clostridium difficile colitis. One patient had nausea and vomiting after laparoscopic radical nephrectomy. The computerized tomography (CT) scan showed mesenteric hernia and the patient underwent internal hernia repair and small bowel resection by open surgery. Another patient who presented with nausea and vomiting because of small bowel obstruction due to adhesions after laparoscopic nephrectomy was treated with lysis of adhesions and small bowel resection by open surgery. One patient who developed acute renal failure, low white blood cell count, and hematemesis after donor nephrectomy was found to have bowel perforation by CT. Open exploration revealed duodenal perforation and the patient was treated by duodenal resection and duodenojejunostomy. Another patient who developed acute renal failure also had abdominal pain after laparoscopic retroperitoneal mass resection after chemotherapy. The patient was evaluated by renal Doppler ultrasonography and MAG-3 renal nuclear scan and diagnosed with thrombosis of right renal artery. Subsequently, open exploration and right nephrectomy was performed. Exploration also revealed a duodenal perforation, which could not be detected by the imaging studies. Duodenal perforation closure was performed. Soulie and coworkers (3) reported a patient who presented with peritonitis 1 week after laparoscopic genital prolapse repair. At open exploration, she had a small perforation of an ileal loop, which was repaired without bowel resection. They also reported two patients with trocar site hernia of ileal loop or cecum after laparoscopic lymph node dissection. One of these patients had signs of bowel obstruction and pain at the unclosed right trocar site 3 days after the primary operation. Incarcerated bowel at the trocar site was detected and repaired by open surgery without bowel resection. The other patient had peritonitis and also pain at the unclosed right trocar site 1 month after the operation. Again, incarcerated bowel at the trocar site was identified and repaired at open exploration without bowel resection. Parra and coworkers (4) reported a patient with perforation of the cecum that was diagnosed 4 days after laparoscopic pelvic lymph node dissection. At open exploration, the findings suggested thermal injury with late rupture and the patient was treated with temporary ileostomy. Another patient became nauseated and showed signs of bowel obstruction 4 days after pelvic lymphadenectomy. Trocar site hernia and incarceration of a loop of ileum through a defect in the fascia at one of the lateral trocar sites was found and treated by the resection of a 12 cm section of midileum and closure of the fascial defect by open surgery. Rassweiler and coworkers (2) reported three patients who underwent reintervention after laparoscopic nephrectomy. Two patients had intestinal stenosis and one patient had trocar site hernia; however, presenting symptoms and the methods of repair were not given. Gill and coworkers (6) reported two patients who developed trocar site hernia after laparoscopic nephrectomy. One of these patients was treated by open and the other by laparoscopic surgery. Eraky and coworkers (7) reported one patient with colonic perforation after laparoscopic nephrectomy, which was managed by open surgery. Kavoussi et al. (8) reported three patients who underwent repeated open surgery due to bowel injury or bowel-related complications after laparoscopic pelvic lymph node dissection. One patient developed rebound tenderness, erythema, and purulent drainage from a trocar site on postoperative day 6. Exploration revealed a small bowel injury, which was oversewn. In one patient, pelvic abscess developed 4 months following node dissection. This patient also had received x-ray therapy to the prostate. At exploration, a small hole was discovered in the sigmoid colon that was repaired. One patient who had small bowel obstruction, which did not resolve with nasogastric suction, required open exploration with excision of a segment of small bowel that had become adherent to the bed of the node dissection. Chow and coworkers (10) reported four patients with bowel-related complications after laparoscopic pelvic lymph node dissection. One patient was treated with open surgery for small bowel obstruction due to adhesions. Another patient who had perforation of sigmoid colon had a CT scan after laparoscopy, which identified pneumoperitoneum but failed to show the perforation. The perforation was found and repaired at open exploration. They also reported two patients with small bowel obstruction due to trocar site hernia. Both were detected by CT scans and underwent subsequent surgical repair.

Urinary leakage is the second most common type of complication that was treated by repeated surgery. Fourteen patients (22.9%) were explored in the postoperative period because of urinary leakage. Yaycioglu and coworkers (5) reported two cases, one of which had abdominal pain and elevated white blood cell count after laparoscopic ureterolithotomy. Computerized tomography scan performed on 15th postoperative day showed pelvic urinoma and abscess formation. The patient was treated with laparoscopic exploration and drainage. The other patient had abdominal pain after laparoscopic pyeloplasty. Computerized tomography scan showed perirenal urinoma and the patient was treated with laparoscopic exploration and nephrostomy tube placement. Soulie and coworkers (3) performed repair by open surgery in one patient because of delayed cutaneous urinary fistula 1 month after laparoscopic resection of hydrocalix. They also reported five patients who were treated by open repair because of disunion of vesicourethral anastomosis 3–10 days after laparoscopic radical prostatectomy (3). Parra and coworkers (4) reported a case that presented with increased abdominal pain, nausea, and occasional emesis 1 month after laparoscopic extended pelvic lymphadenectomy. Computerized tomography scan documented a urinoma over the right iliac vessels. Open surgical exploration revealed a 2 cm segment of the right ureter that was necrotic at the level of the iliac bifurcation. Drainage and reimplantation with a psoas hitch was performed. Kavoussi and coworkers (8) reported two patients who were treated with open surgery due to urinary leakage after laparoscopic pelvic lymph node dissection. One patient developed fever 3 days postoperatively and the CT scan revealed a large urinoma in the pelvis. Open exploration was performed and a transected ureter was repaired. Another patient had bladder injury due to trocar placement. This patient developed hematuria during the node dissection. A postoperative cystogram demonstrated an intraperitoneal rupture. A trial of catheter drainage for 10 days was unsuccessful, open exploration was performed and a perforation at the dome of the bladder was found and repaired. Thomas and coworkers (9) reported a patient who sustained a ureteral injury during laparoscopic pelvic lymph node dissection and was treated by open surgery in the postoperative period. Chow and coworkers (10) reported two patients with ureteral injury after laparoscopic pelvic lymph node dissection. One patient presented with right flank pain 5 weeks after laparoscopic dissection. Computerized tomography scan showed urinary ascites with extravasated urine in the right perinephric and anterior pararenal spaces and also dilatation of the right renal pelvis. Open surgical exploration confirmed the ureteric laceration. Another patient had abdominal distention 3 weeks after laparoscopic dissection. Computerized tomography scan showed multiple cystic collections in the abdomen and right-sided hydronephrosis. Open exploration revealed multiple urinomas and the disruption of right ureter.

Twelve patients (19.7%) underwent repeated exploration because of vascular complications. Yaycioglu and coworkers (5) reported two patients. One had low blood pressure and falling hematocrit levels after laparoscopic donor nephrectomy. Computerized tomography scan showed hematoma of the left rectus muscle and the patient was treated with ligation of inferior epigastric artery by open surgery. The other patient developed acute renal failure and abdominal pain after laparoscopic resection of retroperitoneal mass after chemotherapy. The patient was evaluated by renal Doppler ultrasonography and MAG-3 renal nuclear scan. The patient was diagnosed with thrombosis of right renal artery and underwent subsequent open exploration and right nephrectomy. This patient also had duodenal perforation found at open exploration. Soulie and coworkers (3) performed two emergency reoperations for hemorrhage after radical nephrectomy and varicocelectomy. In both cases, the bleeding was due to misfit of endoscopic clips. Rassweiler and coworkers (2) performed reinterventions to seven cases because of bleeding after laparoscopic nephrectomy. Eraky and coworkers (7) had one case with bleeding from renal vein after laparoscopic nephrectomy that was repaired with open surgery.

Twelve patients (19.7%) had various delayed complications. Rassweiler and coworkers (2) reported four cases of abscess formation and a case of pancreatic fistula after laparoscopic nephrectomy. Gill and coworkers (6) reported two patients who underwent open splenectomy and open surgical resection of duodenal ulcer in the postoperative period because of splenic injury and hemorrhage of a preexisting duodenal ulcer, respectively, after laparoscopic nephrectomy. Also a case of wound dehiscence and a case of perforated diverticulitis treated by open surgery, and three cases of lymphocele formation treated by laparoscopic marsupilization were reported after laparoscopic pelvic lymph node dissection (4,8,9).

Discussion

Delayed bowel complications present with nausea, vomiting, ileus, signs of peritonitis, low white blood cell count, and pain at trocar site with erythema and purulent discharge. However, bowel injuries may also have an atypical presentation. The patient may have persistent pain at a trocar site without erythema or discharge. This finding can be associated with abdominal pain and diarrhea but without leukocytosis, fever, diffuse pain, ileus, nausea, or vomiting. In a retrospective literature review, the average time to recognize a small bowel injury was 4.5 days (range 2–14) and large bowel injury 5.4 days (range 1–29). Thermal injuries presented later than nonthermal injuries (11). Patients with delayed urinary leakage present with signs of infection and the mass effect of the urinoma. These include elevated white cell count, fever, abdominal or flank pain, abdominal distention, nausea, and emesis.

Since clinical findings may be atypical and insufficient for the correct diagnosis, it is advisable to have a low threshold for radiologic evaluation of patients who are acutely ill or symptomatic after urologic laparoscopic surgery. Computerized tomography scan is the best radiologic study and usually reveals the underlying complication accurately. For patients with negative CT scans, management should be planned on an individual basis. Chow and coworkers (10) reviewed the CT findings in their patients with major complications after laparoscopic lymphadenectomy. Clinical evidence of major complications was seen in 12 of 85 patients (14%). Eight of these patients had postoperative abdominal and pelvic examinations and CT findings provided diagnostic information that was used to select appropriate treatment in seven of eight cases. Complications detected on CT scans included small bowel obstruction due to herniation of bowel through the trocar site or to adhesions, hematoma in the abdominal wall, infected retroperitoneal hematoma, urinary ascites or multiple urinomas due to ureteral laceration or transection, and large lymphoceles. In one patient, the CT scan did not reveal the perforation of sigmoid colon. This patient had pneumoperitoneum on CT, which was considered to be due to residual carbon dioxide (CO_2). The bowel, however, appeared normal. Cadeddu and coworkers (12) performed a retrospective analysis in order to determine the indications for and findings of CT in symptomatic patients after urologic laparoscopic surgery. They reviewed data from 400 patients who underwent urologic laparoscopic procedures and identified 20 (5%) who had postoperative symptoms that prompted evaluation by CT scans. They identified 15 complications in 13 patients that were diagnosed by CT. Four patients needed additional interventions for the treatment of pathology that was discovered by CT. Overall, CT made a symptom-related diagnosis in 75% of the time. When performed for a decreasing hematocrit or to evaluate a patient with suspected sepsis CT identified the etiology in 100% of patients. On the other hand, a clear source was identified in only 58% of the time when the CT scan was performed for the evaluation of unexplained flank or abdominal pain. Yaycioglu and coworkers (5) reviewed their experience with patients who underwent repeated exploration within the first month after laparoscopy. Nine patients were treated with repeated exploration from 1226 procedures (0.7%) that were performed within a 7-year period. The symptoms appeared 0–25 days (median 2) after surgery. All patients except one were evaluated by CT scans.

Repeated operations were laparoscopic in four and open in five patients. In all of the patients who were evaluated with CT scan, radiologic findings were consisted with surgical findings and no complications could be identified at exploration that was missed by CT scan. One patient was evaluated by Doppler ultrasonography and renal perfusion scan and a duodenal perforation was undetected which was diagnosed at open exploration.

Once the decision for repeated exploration is made, one has to further decide for the method of exploration. Laparoscopic exploration can be considered especially for patients with persistent symptoms despite negative radiologic studies. Previously, Bauer and coworkers (13) reported their experience with laparoscopy in three postoperative urologic patients with acute abdomen. One of these patients was status post open surgery, other one laparoscopy, and the third was a patient with trauma. They suggested that laparoscopy could provide diagnostic capabilities equivalent to that of open exploration. Laparoscopy is also useful for the drainage of urinomas and the management of lymphoceles (4,5). In other patients, the method of exploration and repair that is appropriate for the diagnosed underlying abnormality should be performed.

ABDOMINAL AIR IN POSTOPERATIVE IMAGING

Free air in the abdomen after laparotomy is a well-recognized phenomenon. It is caused by the room air trapped in the abdominal cavity during wound closure. Laparoscopic surgery is mostly performed by the insufflation of CO_2 into the peritoneal cavity. CO_2 is much more soluble in serum than room air and it is readily excreted from the lungs after it is absorbed by the peritoneum. Therefore, it is expected that pneumoperitoneum after laparoscopy should be smaller in volume and shorter in duration compared to open surgery. Nevertheless, detection of free air in the abdomen at postoperative imaging after laparoscopic procedures is a diagnostic dilemma and

differentiation of its origin should be made. This is especially
true when the patient is being evaluated for postoperative
complications like bowel injury or intraabdominal abscess.
The main sources of abdominal free air after laparoscopic surgery are: pneumoperitoneum due to laparoscopy and abdominal incisions made for hand-assisted laparoscopy or intact
specimen removal, viscus injury, infection with gas forming
organisms, and intraabdominal abscess formation. Other
causes of free air in the abdomen are migration of air into the
abdominal cavity from pneumomediastenum or pneumothorax,
and through the female genital tract (14–16).

   Radiologic studies detect small amounts of free air in
46–70% of the patients 1 day after laparoscopic cholecystectomy in patients without complications. In most of the cases,
free air does not persist for more than a week and the amount
of air decreases with serial radiologic studies. Nonpathologic
free air is usually seen as bubbles located anteriorly adjacent
to the rectus muscles, anterior to the liver and around the trocar sites. However, free air due to bowel perforation can also
be seen as multiple small gas bubbles along the anterior peritoneal surface of the liver. Computerized tomography appearance of air in discrete loculations suggests intraabdominal
infection like infected ascites. The presence of a thickened
colonic wall with paracolonic bubbles is associated with
colonic perforation. In patients who are symptomatic but no
perforation can be demonstrated on imaging, the finding of
increasing amounts of free air and fluid in the abdominal
cavity in repeated CT scans is highly suggestive of an
unrecognized bowel injury.

   McAllister and coworkers (17) obtained upper abdominal
CT scans from 27 consecutive patients approximately 24 hr
after elective laparoscopic cholecystectomy in order to demonstrate postoperative CT findings of uncomplicated laparoscopic cholecystectomy. The majority of the patients were
discharged the day after surgery and no significant postoperative complications occurred. They observed pneumoperitoneum in 19 (70%) patients. The amount of free air was only
several bubbles or a small amount of air located anterior
to the liver, around the position of the previously placed

operative trocars. They found a large amount of free air only in one patient. Five patients (19%) had ascites. The amount of fluid was minimal and usually located in the subhepatic space. In only one patient, there was a moderate amount of fluid. Subcutaneous emphysema was seen in 15 patients (56%). Fourteen of these patients had a minimal amount of subcutaneous emphysema. The authors suggested that since a small amount of pneumoperitoneum is a common finding, only when large or increasing amount of free air are detected should a postoperative complication be considered in the appropriate clinical setting. Also the presence of minimal abdominal fluid following cholecystectomy is well documented and the composition probably consists of serum, blood, lymph, or bile rather than the irrigating solution, which has a low molecular weight and is rapidly absorbed by the peritoneal membrane within 24 hr. The appearance of large or increasing amounts of fluid collections should be viewed with suspicion.

Millitz and coworkers (18) prospectively obtained upright chest radiographs from 50 patients who underwent laparoscopic cholecystectomy on postoperative days 1 (6 hr after surgery), 2, 4, 7, and 14 until the pneumoperitoneum resolved. A perpendicular measurement of any pneumoperitoneum detected between the diaphragm and the liver was made. The pneumoperitoneum was graded as absent, trace (1–5 mm), mild (6–10 mm), or moderate (10–15 mm). None of the patients had any postoperative complications. Pneumoperitoneum was detected postoperatively for various lengths of time in 23 patients (46%). For all but one patient, the pneumoperitoneum resolved in the first week after surgery. In the remaining patient, the pneumoperitoneum resolved in the second week after surgery. The pneumoperitoneum was graded as trace in 17, and mild in six patients. In four patients, the amount of pneumoperitoneum on the second postoperative day radiograph was more extensive than the amount on the first postoperative day. For all the remaining patients, the maximum amount of free air was seen on the initial radiograph. An inverse correlation was detected between body weight and the duration of pneumoperitoneum. Thin patients showed more extensive pneumoperitoneum that lasted longer.

Obese patients, on the other hand, had less extensive pneumo-peritoneum that disappeared sooner. Only 33% of obese patients had pneumoperitoneum postoperatively compared to 62% for thin or average weight patients who had this condition. When the frequency and duration of the pneumoperitoneum was compared with the frequency and duration of pneumoperitoneum reported in the literature for open surgery, the numbers were similar. Since CO_2 should be reabsorbed more quickly than residual room air after laparotomy, it is likely that room air may enter the peritoneal cavity during laparoscopy and this possibly occurs during the insertion and removal of instruments or when a fascial suture is used to close the peritoneal opening. Another explanation is that CO_2 is reabsorbed more slowly than originally anticipated.

Gayer and coworkers (19) investigated the prevalence, duration, and significance of postoperative pneumoperitoneum as detected by CT. They reviewed the 103 postoperative CT examinations of 89 patients who underwent 92 abdominal surgical procedures. Indications for CT were fever and leucocytosis, abdominal pain or distention, suspicious discharge from the drain, general deterioration, vomiting, and wound dehiscence. Prevalence of pneumoperitoneum was 29% after laparotomy and 23% after laparoscopy. The CT scans were performed 1–18 days after surgery. Free air was detected in none of the examinations performed 18–37 days after surgery. Thirteen examinations were performed following laparoscopic procedures. Eight of these were performed within the first 7 days and the other five scans between the 8th and 26th postoperative days. Free air was seen in three scans (23%). In two of these examinations, performed within the first postoperative week, the volume of free air was very small (0.5 and 1 mL). In both cases, the air collected anteriorly, adjacent to the rectus muscles. The third patient had 20 mL of free air 14 days after laparoscopic cholecystectomy. This patient with end-stage renal failure had a moderate amount of ascites secondary to peritoneal dialysis. On CT prior to the laparoscopic surgery, no free air was present. Most of the free intraperitoneal air in this case was in association with the ascites, appearing as discrete loculations containing air–fluid levels, and only about 1 mL was separate from the ascites anterior to the stomach. The patient was reoperated 8 days after CT because of peritonitis, and the ascites proved to be purulent. This was the only patient who had peritoneal intrusion between surgery and CT.

A patient has been reported with peripancreatic retroperitoneal gas mimicking necrotizing pancreatitis after laparoscopic cholecystectomy (20). The patient presented with retroperitoneal gas 7 days after surgery, but did not have the clinical or biochemical features of necrotizing pancreatitis. Resolution of her low-grade fever and of the radiologic findings suggested that the pneumoretroperitoneum was related to the laparoscopic cholecystectomy. Dowdell and coworkers (21) prospectively investigated the prevalence of pneumoperitoneum at CT after laparoscopic cholecystectomy. They obtained CT scans from nine patients within 24 hr of laparoscopic cholecystectomy. They reported that the findings are correlated with duration and difficulty of surgery.

Daly and coworkers (22) reviewed the clinical records of 209 patients who underwent nonbiliary laparoscopic gastrointestinal surgery. Abnormal intraperitoneal gas collections were seen in one patient who had perforation of the colon and pericolonic abscess after retroperitoneal lymph node biopsy for testicular malignancy. The CT scan was performed 3 days after laparoscopic biopsy because of fever. The air was inside a gas containing pericolonic abscess. Abdominal wall gas was detected on CT in four patients as many as 7 days after surgery. In one patient the gas was caused by abscess at a trocar site, and in the remaining three it was caused by postoperative air collections.

Chow and coworkers (10) have previously described a case with sigmoid injury after laparoscopic pelvic lymphadenectomy. The CT scan showed intraperitoneal air but no signs of sigmoid injury.

Cadeddu and coworkers noted intraperitoneal or retroperitoneal gas in four of eight patients who had CT scans within the first week after urologic laparoscopy. Three of these patients had abdominal incisions for specimen retrieval and the fourth case had a perforated ulcer. They suggested that viscus injury should be considered in the appropriate clinical setting when pneumoperitoneum was detected more than 24–48 hr after surgery.

Patients with gastrointestinal perforation are usually detected accurately by CT scan. Jeffrey and coworkers (23) reviewed data from five patients who had clinically unsuspected gastrointestinal perforation and CT evidence of pneumoperitoneum. The clinical indication for obtaining CT scans were blunt abdominal trauma ($n = 2$), suspected pancreatitis ($n = 2$), and possible intraabdominal abscess ($n = 1$). Scans were obtained following both oral and intravenous contrast media. All five patients had CT evidence of pneumoperitoneum. In four cases, multiple small gas bubbles were seen along the anterior peritoneal surface of the liver. In one patient, there was a large hydropneumoperitoneum centrally in the midabdomen. The etiology of the gastrointestinal perforation was demonstrated in four of five patients. This included two patients with perforation of a gastric ulcer which showed extravasation of oral contrast into the lesser sac, one patient with duodenal perforation with paraduodenal gas extending into the right anterior pararenal space as well as pneumoperitoneum, and one patient with colonic perforation which the CT scan revealed a thickened colonic wall and paracolonic gas bubbles. In one patient with a laceration of the jejenum, the site of the perforation was not apparent and the presence of pneumoperitoneum was the only abnormal CT finding.

KEY POINTS

- The repeated exploration rate after urologic laparoscopic surgery is 1.5%.
- Bowel-related, urinary leakage, and vascular complications are the main causes for repeated exploration along with solid organ injuries, lymphocele, and abscess formation.
- Delayed bowel complications present with nausea, vomiting, ileus, signs of peritonitis, low white blood

cell count, and pain at trocar site with erythema and purulent discharge. However, an atypical presentation should also be expected.

- It is advisable to have a low threshold for radiologic evaluation.
- Computerized tomography scan is the first choice of radiologic study.
- Laparoscopic exploration can be considered especially for patients with persistent symptoms despite negative radiologic studies.
- In other patients, the method of exploration and repair that is appropriate for the diagnosed underlying abnormality should be performed.
- Small amounts of free air is found in 46–70% of the patients early after laparoscopic surgery and does not persist for more than a week in most of the cases.
- Computerized tomography appearance of air in discrete loculations suggests intraabdominal infection and the presence of thickened colonic wall with paracolonic bubbles is associated with colonic perforation.
- The finding of increasing amounts of free air and fluid in repeated CT scans is highly suggestive of an unrecognized bowel injury.

REFERENCES

1. Fahlenkamp D, Rassweiler J, Fornara P, Frede T, Loening SA. Complications of laparoscopic procedures in urology: experience with 2407 procedures at 4 German centers. J Urol 1999; 162:765–770.

2. Rassweiler J, Fornara P, Weber M, Janetschek G, Fahlenkamp D, Henkel T, Beer M, Stackl W, Boeckmann W, Recker F, Lampel A, Fischer C, Humke U, Miller K. Laparoscopic nephrectomy: the experience of the laparoscopy working group of the German Urologic Association. J Urol 1998; 160:18–21.

3. Soulie M, Salomon L, Seguin P, Mervant C, Mouly P, Hoznek A, Antiphon P, Plante P, Abbou CC. Multi-institutional study

of complications in 1085 laparoscopic urologic procedures. Urology 2001; 58:899–903.

4. Parra RO, Hagood PG, Boullier JA, Cummings JM, Mehan DJ. Complications of laparoscopic urological surgery: experience at St. Louis University. J Urol 1994; 151:681–684.

5. Yaycioglu O, Ramakumar S, Kavoussi LR, Jarrett TW. Early repeated exploration after laparoscopic urologic surgery: comparison of clinical, radiologic, and surgical findings. Urology 2002; 59:190–194.

6. Gill IS, Kavoussi LR, Clayman RV, Ehrlich R, Evans R, Fuchs G, Gersham A, Hulbert JC, McDougall EM, Rosenthal T, Schuessler WW, Shephard T. Complications of laparoscopic nephrectomy in 185 patients: a multi-institutional review. J Urol 1995; 154:479–483.

7. Eraky I, el-Kappany HA, Ghoneim MA. Laparoscopic nephrectomy: Mansoura experience with 106 cases. Br J Urol 1995; 75:271–275.

8. Kavoussi LR, Sosa E, Chandhoke P, Chodak G, Clayman RV, Hadley HR, Loughlin KR, Ruckle HC, Rukstalis D, Schuessler W, Segura J, Vancaille T, Winfield HN. Complications of laparoscopic pelvic lymph node dissection. J Urol 1993; 149:322–325.

9. Thomas R, Steele R, Ahuja S. Complications of urological laparoscopy: a standardized 1 institutional experience. J Urol 1996; 156:469–471.

10. Chow CC, Daly BD, Burney TL, Krebs TL, Grumbach K, Filderman PS, Jacobs SC. Complications after laparoscopic pelvic lymphadenectomy: CT diagnosis. Am J Roentgenol 1994; 163:353–356.

11. Bishoff JT, Allaf ME, Kirkels W, Moore RG, Kavoussi LR, Schroder F. Laparoscopic bowel injury: incidence and clinical presentation. J Urol 1999; 161:887–890.

12. Cadeddu JA, Regan F, Kavoussi LR, Moore RG. The role of computerized tomography in the evaluation of complications after laparoscopic urological surgery. J Urol 1997; 158:1349–1352.

13. Bauer JJ, Schulam PG, Kaufman HS, Moore RG, Irby PB, Kavoussi LR. Laparoscopy for the acute abdomen in the postoperative urologic patient. Urology 1998; 51:917–919.

14. Gantt CB Jr, Daniel WW, Hallenbeck GA. Nonsurgical pneumoperitoneum. Am J Surg 1977; 134:411–414.

15. Rice RP, Thompson WM, Gedgaudas RK. The diagnosis and significance of extraluminal gas in the abdomen. Radiol Clin North Am 1982; 20:819–837.

16. Winek TG, Mosely S, Grout G, Luallin D. Pneumoperitoneum and its association with ruptured abdominal viscus. Arch Surg 1988; 123:709–712.

17. McAllister JD, D'Altorio RA, Snyder A. CT findings after uncomplicated percutaneous laparoscopic cholecystectomy. J Comput Assist Tomogr 1991; 15:770–772.

18. Millitz K, Moote DJ, Sparrow RK, Girotti MJ, Holliday RL, McLarty TD. Pneumoperitoneum after laparoscopic cholecystectomy: frequency and duration as seen on upright chest radiographs. Am J Roentgenol 1994; 163:837–839.

19. Gayer G, Jonas T, Apter S, Amitai M, Shabtai M, Hertz M. Postoperative pneumoperitoneum as detected by CT: prevalence, duration, and relevant factors affecting its possible significance. Abdom Imag 2000; 25:301–305.

20. Dowdell TR, Leonhardt CM, Arenson AM, Hanna SS. Peripancreatic retroperitoneal gas mimicking necrotizing pancreatitis after laparoscopic cholecystectomy. Can J Surg 1995; 38:547–549.

21. Dowdell TR, Leonhardt CM, Arenson AM, Hanna S. Prevalence of pneumoperitoneum and other gas collections at CT after laparoscopic cholecystectomy: a prospective study. Radiology 1994; 193(suppl):440 (591GI).

22. Daly B, Sukumar SA, Krebs TL, Wong JJ, Flowers JL. Nonbiliary laparoscopic gastrointestinal surgery: role of CT in diagnosis and management of complications. Am J Roentgenol 1996; 167:455–459.

23. Jeffrey RB, Federle MP, Wall S. Value of computed tomography in detecting occult gastrointestinal perforation. J Comput Assist Tomogr 1983; 7:825–827.

14

Medicolegal Issues in Laparoscopic Urology

ROBERT MARCOVICH

Department of Urology,
University of Texas Health
Sciences Center, San Antonio,
Texas, U.S.A.

BENJAMIN R. LEE

Department of Urology,
Long Island Jewish Medical
Center, New Hyde Park,
New York, U.S.A.

INTRODUCTION

Since its introduction in the early 1990s, the laparoscopic approach to urologic surgical problems has benefited innumerable patients through decreased perioperative pain, more rapid recovery, and improved cosmesis. The number of laparoscopic procedures which can be offered to the urologic patient has exploded over the past decade as pioneers have sought to expand the indications for laparoscopy from relatively simple extirpative operations to complex reconstruction.

Despite these beneficial developments, laparoscopy may be associated with a significant risk of medical malpractice litigation (1). Laparoscopy came later to urology than it did to gynecology and general surgery, and as its use increased in the latter disciplines, the risk of medical malpractice litigation also became greater; so much so, that in July 1994 the Association of Trial Lawyers of America founded a Laparoscopic Surgery subgroup to study this emerging area of legal action (2). Numerous articles in the surgical and gynecological literature attempt to address factors that lead to lawsuits in laparoscopic cases, and the insurance industry has also commissioned inquiry into the origins of such litigation (3). The purpose of this chapter is to review the literature on medical malpractice in the realm of laparoscopic surgery, to discuss why the heightened potential for lawsuits relating to laparoscopy exists, and to provide the reader with some general guidelines that may help to decrease the risk of litigation.

CURRENT STATE OF MALPRACTICE IN LAPAROSCOPIC SURGERY

Most of the available information regarding litigation related to laparoscopy comes from the general surgical and gynecological literature. The incidence and prevalence of laparoscopic litigation is difficult to determine. At the 1995 meeting of the Society of Laparoendoscopic Surgery, a survey indicated that 13% of members were occupied with litigation of at least one case involving laparoscopic electrosurgical injury (2). Between 1990 and 1998, there were 40 litigated cases of laparos copic bowel injury closed by the Canadian Medical Protective Association, a nonprofit medical mutual defense organization whose membership includes 95% of licensed Canadian physicians (4).

In 1994, the Physician Insurance Association of America (PIAA)[*] reported a total of 331 claims involving laparoscopic

---

[*]The PIAA is a trade association of over 60 medical malpractice insurance companies, which collectively insure 60% of the private practice physicians in the United States.

cholecystectomy (1), a procedure that was first performed in the United States only 5 years earlier. In comparison, there were 366 claims involving open cholecystectomy cases over the 7-year period from 1985 to 1992. The PIAA found that laparoscopic cholecystectomy litigation was more likely to result in payment to the plaintiff than was open cholecystectomy litigation. In addition to cholecystectomies, the PIAA reported an additional 278 lawsuits related to a variety of laparoscopic procedures, although none were urologic (1). The majority of the other cases comprised diagnostic laparoscopy, tubal ligation, lysis of adhesions, hysterectomy, and salpingo-oophorectomy. Bowel injuries were the most common complications in lawsuits related to the first three procedures, while ureteral and bladder injuries were the most common in the latter two.

In August 2000, the PIAA published results of their laparoscopic injury study (3), which was commissioned as a result of a perceived rapid increase in claims related to laparoscopy. Between 1990 and 1994, 750 claims were filed with PIAA members, while from 1995 to 1999, 1426 claims occurred. Total payout increased from $42 million in the first 5 years to over $104 million during the second 5-year period. In that report, the overwhelming majority of cases were general surgical or gynecological, while only six cases were urological.

MALPRACTICE LITIGATION IN LAPAROSCOPIC UROLOGY

In the spring of 2003, Marcovich and associates (5) at Long Island Jewish Medical Center conducted an internet-based survey of practicing urologists in the United States in order to determine their malpractice histories as related to laparoscopic procedures. Using commercially available software, an e-mail requesting participation in the survey was sent to all active and associate members of the American Urological Association with an e-mail address on file in the society membership directory. Residents, fellows, and nonurologists were excluded. Respondents were initially asked if they perform laparoscopic procedures, and were asked about their training and practice patterns and whether they had been sued over a laparoscopic case. Data were then gathered regarding specific cases up to a total of three per respondent.

Completed surveys were obtained from 426 respondents. Of these, 278 (65.3%) reported performing laparoscopic surgery in their practice for a median number of 3 years (range 1–15 years). By far the largest subset of respondents who were performing laparoscopy had received their training entirely through postgraduate courses only (47.7%). With regard to experience, 200 respondents (71.9%) stated that 10% or fewer of their operative cases were performed laparoscopically, while only 78 (28.1%) did more than 10% of their cases laparoscopically. The median number of laparoscopic cases per year was 15 (range 1–400).

Of the 278 respondents who performed laparoscopy, 19 (6.8%) reported having been sued. Three participants reported two lawsuits and none reported more than two. Of note, there were no statistically significant differences in training and experience profiles of those respondents who were sued in comparison to those who had not been sued. However, a significantly higher percentage of those who were sued reported having extensive laparoscopic experience compared to those who were not sued. The median number of laparoscopic cases performed prior to being sued was 75 (range 10–650 cases). Only five of the respondents sued had done fewer than 50 laparoscopic cases prior to the one which resulted in a claim.

The most common reason for a lawsuit in this survey was an intraoperative injury (15 of 22, 68%); two (9%) cases were due to a nonoperative incident occurring during surgery, three (14%) were related to postoperative occurrences, and two (9%) were classified as "other." The latter included a case of tumor recurrence after laparoscopic nephrectomy and a case of testicular atrophy following laparoscopic orchidopexy. Details of postoperative incidents and nonoperative occurrences during surgery were not sought in the survey.

The majority of claims in this study (13, 59%) were still open, four (18%) had been dropped, three (14%) had settled out of court, and two (9%) had returned a verdict for the urologist. No cases were reported in which a decision had been made in favor of the plaintiff, possibly indicating selection bias. Not surprisingly, some type of nephrectomy was involved in nearly half of the cases. This may be due to the fact that the majority of urological cases currently being performed laparoscopically are renal procedures. The most common surgical approach was pure laparoscopic in 18 (82%); three other cases were performed hand-assisted, and none robotically. In the 15 cases of intraoperative injury, there were 16 structures injured; six (38%) involved the gastrointestinal tract, and half of these were small bowel injuries. No portion of the GI tract was spared, as injuries occurred to stomach, colon, and rectum as well. When taking into account the two bladder injuries, damage to a hollow viscus was the most common form of mishap (eight of 16 cases). Vascular insults occurred in five cases; sites reported were aorta (one), vena cava (one), renal vessels (one), iliac vessels (one) and postoperative hemorrhage following adrenalectomy (one). There was one case of an intercostal nerve injury.

In almost half of the intraoperative injuries, the method causing the insult was sharp dissection (seven of 15, 47%). There were only two cautery injuries and one trocar injury; however, in four of the cases, the device causing injury was unknown. Of the 13 cases in which it would have been possible to recognize the injury intraoperatively, the insult was recognized in only six (46%), most of which were vascular injuries. The majority of insults (five hollow viscus, one nerve, and one vascular) were not recognized at the time of the original procedure; three were recognized and/or repaired within 24 hr and three between 1 and 7 days postoperatively. There was no discernible relationship between outcome of the patient and status of the corresponding claim.

THE RELATIONSHIP BETWEEN LAPAROSCOPY AND MEDICAL MALPRACTICE LITIGATION

There are several important issues when laparoscopy is considered in a medicolegal context. These issues include development of new standards of care, training and certification, and the potential for complications, which may arise and present differently than those in open surgery (6). Neither the importance of communication nor of an appropriately executed informed consent should be underestimated (7).

Standard of Care

Laparoscopy is not a new treatment—it simply represents a new method to deliver established therapy. As such, there is always the potential to compare a laparoscopic operation to an analogous open one, the latter often considered by the medical (and legal) community as the "gold standard." Thus, as the laparoscopic armamentarium is developed, each operation passes through a phase in which it is performed and refined only by a few experts and then, depending on various factors such as the degree of difficulty, reports of efficacy, and the public demand for that type of surgery, it is disseminated with variable penetration into the community.

Therefore, the question of standard of care arises for every laparoscopic procedure. At some point in its evolution, an operation progresses from not being the standard of care to being acceptable. As an example, in 1991 after Clayman and associates (8) reported the first laparoscopic nephrectomy, no one would have argued that removing a cancer-bearing kidney laparoscopically was standard of care, yet that operation was soon to be accomplished, and now laparoscopic radical nephrectomy is universally accepted.

In a field developing as rapidly as laparoscopic urology, this type of evolution has strong implications for medical litigation. When does a laparoscopic procedure become accepted, especially given that open surgical alternatives exist for each one? Is it after the first case report, after the first series is presented, or after its first appearance in a textbook? Unfortunately, there are no clear answers to these questions.

The type of development that laparoscopic operations progress through is illustrated today by the example of laparoscopic partial nephrectomy, which shows that even within the realm of a single procedure, an established standard may be lacking. For example, differences exist in the approaches (pure vs. hand-assisted), the need for hilar clamping, the methods of renal cooling, the techniques used for tumor excision, and the means of obtaining hemostasis. What is the standard method of performing a laparoscopic partial nephrectomy? At this point in time, that question is unanswerable.

Training and Certification

There currently exist no established standards for training or certification of laparoscopic urologists. Fellowship training is certainly an advantage but is probably not necessary for those exposed to a substantial amount of laparoscopy during residency. Certainly, the practitioner should be well versed in the basic principles of laparoscopy, the instrumentation used, how to troubleshoot equipment problems, and the prevention, recognition, and management of intraoperative complications. The learning curve is subjective and differs for various procedures. It has been suggested that the learning curve for laparoscopic nephrectomy is 20 cases, while for laparoscopic prostatectomy it is 50. However, the recent survey of Marcovich and associates (5) on the laparoscopy-related malpractice history of urologists in the United States suggested that experienced laparoscopists are at similar risk of litigation as those who have less experience. It is, therefore, unclear whether the learning curve or the level of training impacts the risk of litigation.

Differences from Open Surgery

The majority of lawsuits stemming from laparoscopic surgery are related to intraoperative injury (1,3,5,6). The techniques of laparoscopy pose a risk for injuries not seen with open surgery, such as needle and trocar injuries to bowel and vasculature. Electrocautery injury to the intestines may occur outside of the surgeon's field of view and may therefore go unrecognized (2). In a series of litigated gynecological cases, Vilos (4) found that 45% of bowel injuries were undetected at the time of injury and these were associated with 67% of the litigation outcomes unfavorable to the surgeon. Both of the PIAA studies confirmed that unrecognized injuries were more likely to result in payment to the plaintiff than recognized injuries (1,3). Marcovich and associates noted that 54% of injuries in their survey went unrecognized, and the majority of these were injuries to the gastrointestinal tract. Those mishaps that were recognized were likely to be vascular (5). Bishoff and coworkers (9) reported that laparoscopic bowel injury presents in a more subtle fashion than open surgical bowel injury, with severe, single trocar site pain, abdominal distention, diarrhea, and leukopenia followed by acute cardiopulmonary collapse secondary to sepsis within 96 hr of surgery. Thus, increased vigilance is necessary both intraoperatively and postoperatively to detect bowel injuries, although evidence suggests that a certain small percentage of bowel injuries will occur despite the most attentive precautions (4). The nature of laparoscopy is such that if a patient does not continually progress after surgery, a complication should be suspected and aggressively sought out (6).

One type of injury that is unique to laparoscopy is the incision that results from conversion to an open procedure. Patients must be made to understand that open conversion can occur in any laparoscopic procedure and he or she should be consented for a possible open operation. The patient should be reassured that conversion to open surgery would only occur for his or her safety or if it is absolutely required in order to meet the goals of the operation. Anecdotal cases exist of patients who have sued their physicians solely because of a conversion to an open procedure, despite an otherwise successful operation, on the basis of disfigurement from a large incision.

Reducing the Risk of Litigation

Can involvement in malpractice litigation be avoided? In a survey of the malpractice histories of urologists listed in "Best Doctors in America," Kaplan reported that 77% of respondents had been sued, with an average of 2.3 claims per urologist. He concluded that there was a direct correlation between time in practice and the risk of being sued, and that professional reputation did not affect the likelihood of being named in a suit (10). This is certainly a dismal outlook that is only worsened by the conclusions of two Harvard School of Public Health studies, which indicated that litigation is ineffective as either a deterrent to negligence or as a compensatory mechanism for patients who have been truly harmed (11,12).

Despite this disheartening evidence, there are precautions that the surgeon can take to decrease the risk of litigation. Doing all that is possible to prevent, recognize, and timely manage complications is of utmost importance. Specific ways to accomplish these three tasks is beyond the scope of this discussion, but some general recommendations will be proposed. First, take the time to ensure that the patient is appropriately positioned and carefully padded in order to avoid a neuromuscular injury, which may complicate an otherwise well-executed operation. Second, always inspect the peritoneal cavity for evidence of needle or trocar injury after access is gained. Neither use of the open Hasson technique nor a visualizing trocar completely eliminates the risk of bowel injury during placement of the primary port (13,14). After placement of the secondary cannula under direct vision, the primary trocar should be inspected with the laparoscope in the secondary port. Third, consider using alternatives to monopolar electrocautery, such as harmonic scalpel or bipolar electrocautery, in order to minimize the risk of organ injury from stray electrical energy (2). Fourth, always assess the completeness of hemostasis at the conclusion of the procedure by reducing the pneumoperitoneum pressure to 5 mmHg. Finally, ensure that the patient is continually improving in the postoperative period. As mentioned previously, lack of progressive improvement after laparoscopy should prompt the surgeon to search for a potential unrecognized injury.

Communication with the patient and family and developing rapport with them are also paramount. Numerous studies show a relationship between the interpersonal aspects of care and the decision to sue a physician (15–17). Levinson and associates (17) found that physicians who educated patients about what to expect, solicited patients' opinions, checked patients' understanding, and encouraged patients to talk, were less likely to have malpractice claims against them. Ambady and coworkers (18) studied the relationship of surgeons' tone of voice to malpractice claims history and found that surgeons who were judged to be more dominant and less concerned or anxious on the basis of their tone of voice were more likely to have been sued than surgeons who were judged to be less dominant and more concerned.

It is advisable, therefore, for the surgeon to take time to educate the patient regarding the disease process for which the laparoscopic procedure is being proposed. This should include a discussion of all the alternatives to laparoscopy, including not operating at all or performing an open procedure. The material risks and benefits of the laparoscopic procedure, of the open alternative, and of not performing surgery at all should be presented. Material risk is defined as a complication that either occurs with a frequency greater than 1% or that a patient would attach reasonable significance to in deciding whether or not to submit to the procedure. It is especially important to inform patients that despite its less invasive nature, laparoscopic surgery still causes pain. For elective cases, which encompass essentially all laparoscopic urologic operations, the patient should be given adequate time to think about the alternatives, discuss them with family members, and think of questions pertaining to the suggested treatment course. The surgeon should be freely available to answer any questions or address any concerns. During lengthy procedures, it may help to reassure the family by a telephone call from the circulating nurse that the operation is progressing well. If a complication does arise, the physician should be open with the patient and family about the occurrence and should be especially attentive to communicating with them and addressing their concerns postoperatively. A patient is more likely to seek legal action if he or she feels abandoned. Ultimately, whether there is a complication or not, the patient should be made to feel that the urologist's overriding goal is his or her well being.

Finally, no discussion of malpractice would be complete without addressing the issue of documentation. The attorney's maxim is that "if it wasn't documented, it wasn't done." All consultations should be noted in writing, and it is especially important to verify that material risks, benefits, and alternatives were discussed and understood. The operative note should indicate all precautions taken to prevent injury and operative findings should be communicated with the patient and family. Batt and McCarthy (7) have suggested that the patient be given copies of intraoperative photographs that demonstrate pertinent findings and correct performance of the procedure, and that such photographs also be placed on the patient's chart. Regardless of the approach, the burden of documentation is carried by the surgeon.

APPENDIX

Checklist to Minimize Risk of Litigation in Laparoscopic Surgery

1. Do the patient and immediate family understand the nature of the disease?
2. Do the patient and immediate family understand the proposed procedure? Diagrams and printed literature are very effective ways to communicate this.
3. Have they been given alternatives to the procedure, including a discussion of the risk of not undergoing it?
4. Have they been informed of the material risks of the procedure?
5. Do they understand that open conversion may be necessary to complete the procedure in the most efficacious and safe way possible?
6. Has the surgeon made the patient understand that he/she is concerned for the safety and well being of the patient?
7. Has the surgeon given the patient and family ample opportunity to think about the treatment course and addressed their questions and concerns?
8. Does the surgeon feel confident that his training and experience will allow successful execution of the procedure?

9. Does the surgeon understand how to prevent, recognize, and treat the unique complications associated with laparoscopic surgery?

10. Has the surgeon been vigilant in

- ensuring proper positioning and padding of the patient?
- searching meticulously for abdominal entry injuries before beginning the operation?
- minimizing the use of monopolar electrocautery?
- assessing for satisfactory hemostasis prior to exiting the abdomen?

11. Is the surgeon satisfied that the patient is continually progressing in the postoperative period?

REFERENCES

1. Physician Insurers Association of America. Laparoscopic Procedure Study, Rockville, MD, 1994.

2. Perantinides PG, Trarouhas AP, Katzman VS. The medicolegal risks of thermal injury during laparoscopic monopolar electrosurgery. J Healthcare Risk Manage 1998; 18:47–55.

3. Physician Insurers Association of America. Laparoscopic Injury Study, Rockville, MD, 2000.

4. Vilos GA. Laparoscopic bowel injuries: forty litigated gynaecological cases in Canada. J Obstet Gynaecol Can 2002; 24:224–230.

5. Marcovich R, Rastinehad A, El-Hakim A, Smith AD, Lee BR. Medical malpractice trends in contemporary urological laparoscopy: results of an Internet survey. J Urol 2004; 171(suppl):127.

6. Rein H. Complications and litigation in gynecologic endoscopy. Curr Opin Obstet Gynecol 2001; 13:425–429.

7. Batt RE, McCarthy JV. Communication and documentation before and after laparoscopic surgery. J Am Assoc Gynecol Laparosc 1999; 6:379–381.

8. Clayman RV, Kavoussi LR, Soper NJ, et al. Laparoscopic nephrectomy. N Engl J Med 1991; 324:1370–1371.

9. Bishoff JT, Allaf ME, Kirkels W, Moore RG, Kavoussi LR, Schroder F. Laparoscopic bowel injury: incidence and clinical presentation. J Urol 1999; 161:887–890.

10. Kaplan GW. Malpractice risks for urologists. Urology 1998; 51:183–185.

11. Localio AR, Lawthers AG, Brennan TA, et al. Relation between malpractice claims and adverse events due to negligence: results of the Harvard Medical Practice Study III. N Engl J Med 1991; 325:245–251.

12. Brennan TA, Sox CM, Burstin HR. Relation between negligent adverse events and the outcomes of medical-malpractice litigation. N Engl J Med 1996; 335:1963–1967.

13. Sadeghi-Nejad N, Kavoussi LR, Peters CA. Bowel injury in open technique laparoscopic cannula placement. Urology 1994; 43: 559–560.

14. Thomas MA, Rha KH, Ong AM, et al. Optical access trocar injuries in urological laparoscopic surgery. J Urol 2003; 170: 61–63.

15. Beckman HB, Markakis KM, Suchman AL, Frankel RM. The doctor patient relationship and malpractice—lessons from plaintiff depositions. Arch Intern Med 1994; 154:1365–1370.

16. Hickson GB, Clayton EW, Entman SS, et al. Obstetricians' prior malpractice experience and patients' satisfaction with care. JAMA 1994; 272:1583–1587.

17. Levinson W, Roter DL, Mullooly JP, Dull VT, Frankel RM. Physician-patient communication. The relationship with malpractice claims among primary care physicians and surgeons. JAMA 1997; 277:553–559.

18. Ambady N, LaPlante D, Nguyen T, Rosenthal R, Chaumeton N, Levinson W. Surgeons' tone of voice: a clue to malpractice history. Surgery 2002; 132:5–9.

Index